THE MANPOWER PROBLEM
IN MENTAL HOSPITALS

THE MANPOWER PROBLEM IN MENTAL HOSPITALS

A Consultant Team Approach

PHILIP F. D. SEITZ, M.D., ELIZABETH JACOB, M.S.W.,
HAROLD KOENIG, M.D., PH.D, RUTH KOENIG, M.D.,
WARREN G. MCPHERSON, M.D., ARTHUR A. MILLER, M.D.,
ROBERT L. STEWART, M.D., and
DOROTHY STOCK WHITAKER, PH.D.

INTERNATIONAL UNIVERSITIES PRESS, INC.
New York

Library of Congress Cataloging in Publication Data
Main entry under title:

The Manpower problem in mental hospitals.

    Bibliography: p.
    Includes index.
1. Psychiatric consultation. 2. Psychiatric
hospitals—Employees—In-service training.
3. Psychiatric hospital care—Bibliography.
I. Seitz, Philip F. D.
RC455.2.C65M36   616.8'91   76-18935
ISBN 0-8236-3142-7

Manufactured in the United States of America

Contents

∽❧∾

Acknowledgments

The members of the Chicago consultant team express their appreciation to those who aided them in this project: Drs. Harold M. Visotsky and Francis J. Gerty, Former Directors, Illinois Department of Mental Health; Drs. Robert C. Drye and Jules H. Masserman, Former Directors of Education, Illinois State Psychiatric Institute; Dr. Lester H. Rudy, Former Superintendent, Illinois State Psychiatric Institute; Dr. Percival Bailey, Former Executive Secretary, The Illinois Research and Training Authority;[1] Dr. Gerhart Piers, Director Emeritus, Chicago Institute for Psychoanalysis; The Board of Mental Health Commissioners, State of Illinois; Dr. Galvin Whitaker, who helped in developing the form and concept of Chapter VI; Mrs. Dorothy Huffman, our original Administrative Assistant; Mrs. Gene Knop, who carried on as Administrative Assistant for most of the Midwest project and all of our second state hospital project; Mrs. Trudy Rafelson, the project's hard-working secretary; Mrs. Kate Ollendorff, our Editorial Assistant. Funds for publication of the book were contributed by

[1]The project was supported in large part by a grant from the Illinois Research and Training Authority.

the Ritter Foundation, New York City. We would add special acknowledgment and salute to the staff and patients at Midwest State Hospital, and to the Illinois City Consultant Team.[2]

[2]The names of the hospital, its staff, and the members of the Illinois City Consultant Team have been changed in order to make this report as candid and accurate as possible.

Preface

With the advent of psychotropic drugs, the doors of mental hospitals began to open. Increasing numbers of patients could be returned to the community and maintained there. An unfortunate, ironic consequence of this change, however, has been that mental hospitals and their patients, hitherto always neglected by the medical profession, politicians, and the public, now receive even less attention, less professional help, and less financial support than before.

The initial popularity of Community Psychiatry appears to have peaked during the past decade (1965-1975) and begun to decline. As the public became aware of Community Psychiatry and some of its consequences — especially the increasing numbers of mentally ill in the community and the frequent impossibility of hospitalizing those who were very disturbed — voices of opposition began to be heard. A recent article by Mark Vonnegut asked:* "If hospitalization is such a dreadful thing, one wonders why the rich are still using it, and letting the poor have such a marvelous new system of maintenance

---

*Reprinted by permission from *Harper's Magazine,* February, 1975, © 1975.

in the community. Hospitalization—getting the hell out of the community, the family, the job—is often an essential part of getting well."

Vonnegut proposed that more adequate studies be made of recently discharged mental patients and that wholesale discharges of such patients be stopped: "It is essential that Community Mental Health not be carelessly unleashed on the public; it should be tested as carefully as if it were a new drug."

Some recent studies of the type Vonnegut suggested have produced a storm of controversy among mental health professionals. A recent investigation by Zitrin revealed that arrests, including arrests for crimes of violence, are significantly higher in patients admitted to and discharged from mental hospitals than for others in the community. In another such study, H. B. M. Murphy of McGill University found that, although foster home placements of the mentally ill are increasing steadily, they show no clinical advantages over hospital care in reducing chronicity and promoting normalcy. Rather than increasing normal behavior, according to Murphy, the effects of foster home care appeared to be largely in "reducing active behavior": "This 'improvement' can be described as a shift toward passivity, characterized by loss of vigor, determination, inner drive, and interests."

In this connection, both public and professional concern is now being expressed about abuse of discharged mental patients by operators of boarding homes. The *New York Times*, on March 15, 1975 (p. 32) reported cases of discharged mental patients having been chained, beaten, and carried against their will to remote housing facilities in the country. The boarding-home operators were charged with kidnapping. A Philadelphia psychiatrist, W. L. Clovis, observed about such abuses: "We have forgotten some basic facts in the rush to protect everyone from 'snakepits,' which were considered somehow intrinsically evil because of their large size and distant location. Some patients are so ill that they need varying degrees of protection for the rest of their lives, and some can only use custodial care...We have also forgotten that many of the problems of state hospitals were caused because society silently but deliberately chose not to fund real treatment and not to provide much in the way of humane care for long-term patients."

Despite the promises of Community Psychiatry to close down mental hospitals, these venerable institutions are still with us and likely to remain. The authors of this book, facing that fact, concluded that if mental hospitals were to remain with us they should be improved. The question was, How?

The most serious single problem of large mental hospitals is a shortage of manpower—not only in numbers, but, even more important, in the skills and effectiveness of the hospital staff and personnel. The traditional approach to manpower problems in large mental hospitals by recruitment methods—including "piracy" of personnel from other hospitals and states—does not solve the problem. It merely moves the existing pool of personnel around from one understaffed hospital to another.

The approach we have developed over a period of six years at two large mental hospitals attempts to deal with the manpower problem by improving the morale, the clinical skills and effectiveness of *existing personnel* at such hospitals through systematic and coordinated training programs. Urban specialists in the medical and social sciences join together as a teaching team — a small faculty — for a geographically remote mental hospital and, over a period of several years, provide integrated training programs for the entire staff and personnel of that hospital.

The methods and effectiveness of the first such three-year project are described in this book. The success of the consultant-team approach is demonstrated by its results.

Despite the difficulties of commuting to a hospital two hundred miles from Chicago, all of the consultants found the work so stimulating and rewarding that they continued the project for the entire three years, and most of them went on to commute to a second state hospital for another three years. Their morale and enthusiasm for the project were such that every week, for the entire three years, regardless of weather or other contingencies, one or more of the consultants arrived at the hospital for a full day of teaching.

The training programs generated so much interest and enthusiasm among the hospital staff and personnel that their morale, skills, and effectiveness in working with mental patients, and also their commitment to the hospital, increased steadily during the three years of the project. In contrast to the usual rapid turnover of staff and personnel in such hospitals, the hospital in which we worked developed the most stable staff in the entire state hospital system of Illinois.

Moreover, the clinical skills and confidence of the staff improved so much that increasing numbers of patients were transferred to the hospital from overcrowded hospitals in the metropolitan Chicago area. The admission rate more than doubled by the third year of the project. The discharge rate from the hospital rose to ninety-four per cent by the third year of the project—an increase of more than twenty per cent.

Psychiatrists in communities near the hospital became so interested in what we were doing—having previously avoided the hospital—that they formed a consultant team of their own on the model of the Chicago team, worked with the Chicago team during the third year of the project, and continued the training programs themselves for another four years after the Chicago consultants left.

The results of the second project—not described in the present volume—further confirmed the effectiveness of this approach to the manpower problems of large mental hospitals.

It is our hope that the story of our experience will interest other urban specialists and other mental hospitals in the consultant team approach.

❧

CHAPTER ONE

The Consultant Team

TRAVELING PSYCHIATRIC CONSULTANTS have long been a part of the welfare scene in Illinois, and a good many psychiatrists have at one time or another made trips from Chicago to the large state institutions lying to the west and south of the city. There, in an effort concentrated into a single day, perhaps once a month, they have attempted to teach dynamic psychiatry to a more or less untrained staff responsible for from one to five thousand mentally disturbed patients. Visits of this nature have necessarily been limited to formal lectures for the medical staff with occasional visits to the wards for diagnostic and other clinical teaching purposes.

It was an invitation to become such an occasional consultant to a hospital of his choice that caught the imagination of our project's coordinator and led to the formation of the Chicago Consultant Team.

He was aware of the frustrations that would meet the efforts of any single commuting teacher, but he was equally convinced of the overwhelming need for devoted and experienced consultants within the state hospital system. It occurred to him that a *group* of psychoanalysts, analytically trained psychologists, and social workers,[1] banded together as a coordinated team of consultant teachers, might, over a period of several years, have a real and lasting effect upon a geographically isolated state hospital. Such a team would of necessity speak the same professional language (which for our group was psycho-analysis); the members would also need mutual respect, a shared enthusiasm for the project, and a workable system of communication—probably through the headquarters of a team-member coordinator.

Coincidence also played a part in the consultant team's development: the Illinois Department of Mental Health announced plans to increase the number of, and stipends for, psychiatric consultants to Illinois state hospitals. State support for a consultant team thus became available at the same time that the idea was conceived. A proposal was quickly drafted and submitted to the appropriate state authorities. We reproduce it.

Purpose of this proposal

In the proposed statewide extension of the State Hospital Training Program, which is designed to raise the level of patient care in state hospitals, a special need has been expressed for consultants who are willing to devote a full day of teaching and service, once or twice monthly throughout the year, at a state hospital of their choice. The idea has occurred to me that if a

---

[1]The consultant team for the second state hospital project also included two psychiatric nurse consultants. Neurologists were also attached to both consultant teams.

group of four or five psychoanalysts, a neurologist, a psychologist, and a psychiatric social worker would band together as a team of consultants to a particular state hospital of their choice, each agreeing to spend one day a month at the hospital, a more substantial and better organized program of teaching and service could be provided for that hospital. If the members of such a team would rotate their visits to the hospital, the hospital would have at least one consultant regularly one full day each week. If the group of consultants were organized as an integrated team, a coordinated program of teaching, research, and service could be planned to make the fullest and most effective use of the consultants' respective interests, talents, and time. I am interested in attempting to organize such a team on a trial or experimental basis.

Tentative plans for such a project

First, it would be necessary to recruit three or four other psychoanalysts as well as a neurologist, psychologist, and psychiatric social worker. Preferably, and if possible, these should be colleagues selected largely on the basis of their compatibility as a working team.

Choice of a hospital

I would favor a hospital with the following characteristics: first, a hospital in the greatest need of such help. Since the state hospitals near metropolitan centers have less difficulty in attracting consultants, the hospital selected for this project should probably be downstate and somewhat isolated geographically and thus professionally. In addition, the hospital should be one that desires a program of this kind, and has at least some doctors, psychologists, and psychiatric social workers who are fairly eager and also qualified for further training. From my inquiries, Midwest State Hospital might fit these criteria rather well.

General orientation or philosophy of this project

It is assumed that most of the doctors in the state hospitals are already fairly familiar with the organic psychiatric approach and therapies.[2] It seems likely, therefore, that the greatest need is for further training and experience in psychological dynamics, i.e., knowledge and skills that help the doctor discover and understand the individual patient's particular personality problems, his characteristic patterns of dealing with those problems, and the factors in his development that produced the problems and defense mechanisms. It is not assumed that training and service of this kind would necessarily produce any great change in the number of patients helped to leave the hos-

---

[2]Even this assumption of a basic psychiatric skill on the part of the hospital staff turned out to be incorrect.

pital.[3] The general orientation or philosophy of this project would be more along the lines stated in the aims of the state training program announcement, viz. "to raise the level of patient care." A project of this kind would attempt to promote better patient care by its emphasis upon understanding the individual patient.

General strategy of the team's approach

One of the most important functions of such a team would be that of stimulating and inspiring professional enthusiasm and therapeutic hope among the doctors and other personnel of the hospital. Elevation of the doctors' morale alone might affect the therapeutic atmosphere of the entire hospital. Enthusiasm of this kind could not possibly be sparked simply by lectures or the teaching of abstract concepts. More impressive and tangible approaches would be needed, particularly direct participation of the consultants in clinical work with patients. Since many of the patients in the hospital are there for long periods of time, it would be possible for a consultant to interview certain patients repeatedly each time he returned for another monthly visit. The gradually deepening understanding of these patients by the doctors being trained, and their growing

[3]This assumption turned out to be overly modest: by the end of the three-year project, the discharge rate had increased by twenty per cent.

identification with the patience, skill, and therapeutic attitudes of the consultants, could inspire new hope and enthusiasm in the doctors for their difficult and often discouraging work.

Another aspect of the team's general strategy would be that of organizing research projects. Immediately tangible therapeutic results often are not possible in severely ill hospitalized patients. Discouragement among the personnel caring for such patients can sometimes be lessened by a more investigative attitude toward the problems. The research projects themselves could be quite modest ones, with very limited goals. Their primary purpose would be to encourage and inspire an investigative interest in an approach to some of the difficult problems of state hospital psychiatry. "Action research" projects also might be undertaken, e.g., single wards might be selected for experiments in group therapy, patient government, work with patients and aides alone, etc. The consultant team would attempt to get underway at the hospital as many research projects as possible, and to give active and direct assistance and supervision in the design, planning, carrying-out, writing-up, and publication of such researches.

A final strategic approach would be that of teaching a body of theoretical knowledge about personality dynamics and development, which would give the doctors (and other staff persons) a feeling of gratification and confidence in having acquired and mastered a valuable new intellectual possession and tool. This program of teaching should involve as much active participation as possible on the part of the staff—in contrast to more passive methods of learning through lectures, etc. This policy could be implemented by various teaching devices, such as "home work" between teaching sessions, reports by the staff on assigned topics, and by encouraging the staff to organize additional teaching programs for themselves and for other hospital personnel.

Specific plans and "tactics"

This is not the time to spell out the details of such a program, since whatever programs might be designed should be tailored to fit the needs of the individual hospital, its doctors, and other staff groups. It should be based upon the particular interests, talents, and time of the psychoanalysts and other professionals recruited for the consultant team. The first function of such a team would be to visit the hospital selected, get acquainted with the doctors, other persons, and problems there, and then begin a series of meetings with each other and with the hospital staff to hammer out a workable program.

The morale, enthusiasm, and hope of the consultant team would be an important factor in its effectiveness. To that end, the team would need a great deal of freedom and also support from the Psychiatric Training and Research

Authority of the State of Illinois. If the project were effective in one hospital, then, after operating in that hospital for two or three years, the team could be shifted to other hospitals where its work might be needed and useful.

If possible, an attempt should be made to interest the psychiatrists in the hospital's nearby communities in forming a consultant team to replace the Chicago team after three years. The local psychiatrists could continue and extend the clinical, training, and research programs initiated by the Chicago team. They would constitute a maintenance force of consultants for the hospital after the Chicago team had completed its intensive training program.

Many of the goals and methods of the project as it actually developed were anticipated in the original proposal. Both the plan and Midwest as the selected hospital were approved by the State authorities. The necessary financial support for the consultant team was allocated with minimal delay. Funds for the administrative office and staff of the project were provided by the Illinois Research and Training Authority; consultants' fees and travel expenses were paid for by the Department of Education, Illinois State Psychiatric Institute.

The official hurdles cleared, the coordinator turned to the task of recruiting the team. Knowing that the entire plan could collapse at this crucial point, he turned at once to colleagues he knew well, both professionally and personally, and issued invitations to Drs. Robert L. Stewart and Warren G. McPherson, psychiatrists with whom he had worked closely for years before at the Indiana University Department of Psychiatry. In addition, he sought the help of Dr. Harold Koenig, Professor of Neurology at Northwestern University; Miss Elizabeth Jacob, then Chief Psychiatric Social Worker at the Institute for Psychoanalysis; and Dr. Dorothy Stock, psychologist in the Department of Psychiatry at the University of Chicago. Although some members of the team had not known each other previously, all had fairly extensive and intimate working contact with Dr. Philip Seitz, the coordinator of the group.[4]

Responding promptly, all five indicated their interest in the project as outlined, and the core of the commuting team was established. Within days, Mrs. Dorothy Huffman joined the team in the essential position of Administrative Assistant with responsibility for team communication and all administrative and secretarial details (a position later filled by Mrs. Gene Knop). An additional psychiatric consultant, Dr. Ruth Koenig, later joined the team, bringing to the project considerable previous experience in state mental hospitals and interest in the hospital as an organization; and toward the end of the first year, still another psychoanalyst, Dr. Arthur Miller (deceased), was added to the consultant team, partially in response to the Nursing Staff's request for consultation. These ten professionals, plus the Administrative Assistant and a secretary, constituted the Chicago consultant team to Midwest State Hospital.

The consultant team visited the hospital together only one time as a group. Unfortunately, no allowance

---

[4]The question has been raised of how great a role the personality of the coordinator played in the original formation and consolidation of the team. That it played some part is undeniable, but it should not be assumed that this was a major factor in the motivation of the group. It is almost certain that those who joined were motivated primarily by interest in the idea and by the possibilities of the project, rather than by personal ties to the coordinator.

was made for a series of introductory meetings with the hospital administration and staff. Using that most irritating of measures, hindsight, this was a mistake and led to some weaknesses in the project. Had the consultant team been less rushed and eager to begin its work, there might have been a period of collaborative planning with the hospital, which in turn would have involved the staff and administration more deeply in the plans from the outset. As it was, the project simply commenced, based more upon enthusiasm and hope than upon carefully detailed policies and plans. The result was insufficient preparation of the hospital personnel and inadequate working formulas for the guidance of staff and consultants. It should be noted that this situation was corrected when the team began its second project at another state hospital. The consultants spent almost a year on initial planning and individual visits with the hospital staff before the second project actually started.

The earliest contact with the hospital staff was made by the coordinator on his first reconnaissance visit to the hospital. The impressions gained on that trip laid the groundwork for many of the subsequent goals and working procedures of the project. Perhaps the most important of his impressions was the great need of the medical staff for clinical guidance in dealing with patients. "We don't know what to do with psychiatric patients; come tell us," summarized their response to queries about how the consultants might help. Anxiety among the doctors about their lack of psychiatric knowledge and skills, as well as outright fear of the patients, was evident, and the alleviation of this anxiety became a major goal of the project. In his first memorandum to the consultants suggesting approaches to their teaching task, the coordinator outlined some possible remedies for the situation: (a) sharing responsibility with the doctors for difficult clinical decisions; (b) using the preceptor system in teaching; (c) extending clinical support to cover the time between visits by encouraging phone calls to Chicago when necessary; (d) lessening fear by letting the doctors observe the consultants working with disturbed patients; and (e) encouraging discussion of their fears during individual conferences with preceptors.

The lack of confidence on the part of the medical staff concerning psychiatric problems, so apparent to the coordinator, was also visible to the other staff groups within the hospital; clearly, methods would have to be found to deal effectively and tactfully with this imbalance. We decided to have closed conferences with the doctors, which would be attended only by the psychologist and social worker directly involved with the patient under discussion. The consultants adopted a related policy of being as discreet as possible in any talks with the doctors that involved the other disciplines.

Planning for the project was continued at a collaborative meeting of the staff and consultant team at the hospital. This meeting covered general principles as well as specific plans for the team's work at the hospital, as noted in the following trip report:

Following a short sight-seeing tour of the Midwest community, the team met for two hours with Dr. Gordon (Superintendent), Dr. Lester Rudy of the Illinois State Psychiatric Institute, and the various department heads of the hospital. The discussion covered both general principles of, and specific plans for, the team's work at the hospital

One of the general principles established at this meeting was that the psychiatrists and neurologist of the team would work primarily with the staff physicians, rather than with psychologists, social workers, or other professional personnel. This policy was considered necessary in order to help the staff doctors develop a professional identity as psychiatrists and eventually professional leadership in the hospital as physicians trained in psychiatry.

Another general principle agreed upon was that the training of the staff physicians would be done primarily by the apprentice system rather than by emphasizing didactic instruction. Each of the psychiatric consultants would become the principal supervisor for three or four of the staff doctors—although the doctors would have contact and consultations with all of the consultants.

The possibility of enlisting additional consultant services from psychiatrists in nearby communities was discussed. Dr. Seitz agreed to make inquiries about the experience and qualifications of such psychiatrists and to bring the matter up again later for consideration by the hospital administration and the consultant team.

Friday was decided upon as the day for visits by the consultants, and each consultant would visit the hospital on one Friday every month. Every effort should be made to maintain a regular schedule of such visits. In bad weather, if traveling were impossible on a certain day, the consultant for the week should not simply cancel his visit, but should arrange with the hospital to come on an alternative day. When a holiday fell on Friday, the consultant for that week should come on Thursday or some other day of the same week. The four men consultants agreed to rotate their weekly visits, the two women consultants making one visit apiece per month, accompanying one of the men.

The Acting Clinical Director at the hospital should coordinate the appointments and schedules of the staff doctors for their conferences, individual meetings, and seminars with the consultants. He would select the cases for teaching staff conferences, and supervise the preparation and work-up of cases for these conferences.

The following tentative plans were made about how the consultants' time would be allocated:

Psychiatric consultants

Morning schedule. Teaching staff conference, all staff physicians attending. One or two cases to be staff thoroughly. The staff doctor should present his history and mental examination; the consultant would interview the patient; the psychological and social service reports would be reviewed, and ample time given to discussing the case and the problems it presents.

Afternoon schedule. Individual conferences with staff doctors about problem cases, etc.

On Dr. Stock's monthly visits, a seminar on ward milieu and patient government.

End of the afternoon: Seminar on basic psychiatry, coordinated by the three psychiatric consultants.

Tentative plans about sequence of subjects and references for first year of this seminar:

Bosselman, B. C.: *Neurosis and Psychosis.* Springfield, C. C Thomas, 1950. (Organic syndromes to be covered by Dr. Koenig.)

Section on psychodynamics in: Noyes, A. P.: *Modern Clinical Psychiatry.* Philadelphia, Saunders, 1958.

Colby, K. M.: *Primer for Psychotherapists.* N. Y., Ronald Press, 1951.

Neurological consultant

Morning schedule. Formal staffing of three or four neurological patients worked up in advance, all staff physicians attending.

End of morning: Informal discussion of questions and problems.

Afternoon schedule. Class on clinical neurology. Informal ward rounds on neurological cases.

End of afternoon: Class on basic neurology.

Psychological consultant

Morning schedule. Because some of the psychologists will be at the psychiatric staff conferences and Dr. Stock will also attend some of these conferences, her morning time will be used for individual conferences with members of the psychology staff.

Afternoon schedule. Seminars on group therapy.

(a) Seminar on general problems that arise in group therapy.

(b) Case seminar using tapes of therapy sessions.

(c) Seminars on ward milieu and patient government (for staff doctors).

Psychiatric social work consultant

Plans and schedules to be worked out collaboratively with Chief Psychiatric Social Worker and Staff.

It is interesting to note, on looking back, that the details worked out at this early date actually stamped the final character of the Midwest project and that such changes as were made fitted by and large into the original outline.

The final phase of advance planning took place on the return trip to Chicago, with the consultants agreeing on methods of intrateam communication. There would be a monthly breakfast meeting of the entire group for discussion of seminar curricula, future plans, and problems. Following each consultant's visit to the hospital, he would dictate a summary of his experience, and these reports would be transcribed by the team secretary and circulated immediately by the administrative assistant to all team members. The coordinator would also telephone each departing and returning consultant to keep informed of all developments and to pass along last-minute information that might prove useful at the hospital.

All of the general principles mentioned in the foregoing pages were proposed by the consultant team and concurred in by the hospital staff after brief discussion. The only actual *collaborative* planning with the staff revolved around the curriculum and the allocation of the consultants' time at the hospital, with most of the suggestions about these matters emanating from the staff.

Mention should perhaps be made of some areas of discussion that were conspicuous by their absence in these first meetings. One was any arrangement for regular meetings between the consultants and the Superintendent. Another was the establishment of procedures for written communication between consultants and hospital staff; the consultants were naïvely unaware that this hospital was one (of many) requiring that all such messages filter through the Superintendent's office. Both of these omissions were later corrected, and arrangements were made for each consultant's schedule to include a meeting with the Superintendent and for consultants and staff to exchange notes freely, although a copy of each such memorandum was still to be sent to the front office. The stage, if not ideally set for collaboration and smooth functioning, was at least chalked out in advance of the first consultant's first teaching visit to the hospital.

CHAPTER TWO

The Hospital

THE MIDWEST STATE HOSPITAL is only one of thirteen state hospitals within the Illinois system, but in several ways it was the most logical choice for the first experiment in team teaching.

Although far enough from Chicago to be relatively isolated from its psychiatric training programs and libraries, the hospital and nearby Illinois City are still only two hundred miles from Chicago and linked to it by a major airline, by rail, and by a moderately good highway. Commuting to this area is, making due allowance for winter storms, a relatively easy matter.

Midwest State Hospital was attractive to us because of its prevailing atmosphere of progress and its willingness to try out new ideas. Before the advent of the consultant team, Dr. Gordon, Superintendent of the hospital, had not only expressed a wish for psychiatric consultants, but, several years before, had already negotiated with a nearby university and college for consultants and teachers for his staff. To be sure, the wish for outside consultants contained undertones of ambivalence, which became

17

more apparent as the strangers moved into and through the hospital. But these feelings were not clearly apparent at the start of the project, nor were they surprising for so complex and established an institution.

Another example of progress was the fact that the hospital had already opened most of its previously locked doors; the Superintendent had succeeded in removing the locks from all but ten per cent of the tight-security wards. This advance was due in part, no doubt, to the use of psychopharmacologic agents. In some aspects, chemical restraints had been substituted for physical ones, although the open wards indicated a strong current of progress moving within the institution.

In other ways, too, Midwest had been making a determined effort to treat its patients along more progressive lines. Although geared to offer little more than custodial care to its eighteen hundred patients, the hospital was struggling to reach beyond its custodial function toward offering more dynamic therapies designed to rehabilitate patients and return them to the community. An extensive Family Care Program was evidence of this progressive tendency. But other efforts toward a dynamic approach were severely hampered by the lack of an adequate psychiatric staff.

It is often said that understaffing is the big problem confronting state hospitals today, but Midwest demonstrated that the problem may even be a total *lack* of psychiatric staff. At the beginning of the project, there were ten ward physicians at the hospital, none of whom had any training whatsoever in psychiatry. The Superintendent had had some training in psychiatry, but he was so tied down with administrative responsibilities that he could not provide professional psychiatric guidance to his staff. An additional anomaly was that, in a relatively prosperous and more or less ethnically homogeneous area of the rural United States, not one of the ten doctors was native born. Indeed, they represented a United Nations in microcosm, coming from the Philippines, Poland, Lithuania, Greece, Germany, Yugoslavia, Mexico, Cuba, and Colombia. These facts alone have far-reaching implications about the social structure of the hospital, including its caste system—which is an integral part of any such institution.

The first impression made by a vast state hospital is almost always a forceful and sometimes an unforgettable one. Even for the professional team of consultants, all of whom had had previous experience in psychiatric hospitals, the first day at Midwest had a lasting impact. As they approached the hospital, they were greeted by a complex of castles on the Rhine topped with decorative stone gingerbread. The castles, however, had been neglected to the point of decay, and the gingerbread was becoming something of a hazard to the passer-by— enough to cause its removal a year or two later.

Within, the buildings were fairly clean and livable, although drab and overcrowded. The patients themselves seemed physically well cared for, and on the summery day of the first visit they were moving about the grounds freely and the little supervision they were being given was unobtrusive. But the visitors found the atmosphere oppressive and depressing. Patients passed each other and the members of the consultant team without betraying a flicker of human recognition or interchange. In the Occupational Therapy shop, the patients were engaged in tasks of a manual, repetitive nature, and working in the same withdrawn and isolated way. One consultant later recalled having been struck by a feeling of physical coldness on that first visit to the hospital, despite the warmth and sunniness of the day. The consultants found themselves turning to each other for the contact that seemed so conspicuously lacking among the patients, a reaction that may have had an important unifying effect upon the team.

Like most state hospitals, Midwest was arranged so that all of the intensive diagnostic and treatment work was done in one building, known as the Admissions Building. It had three floors, of which the first and third were open, the middle one locked. On each floor were two wards, men in one and women in the other. Every one of the six wards had twenty-five beds, so that the entire unit had seventy-five male and seventy-five female patients. Inasmuch as all the other wards were "chronic," it was agreed that the consultants should concentrate on the Admissions Building where they would also have available an interviewing suite with a one-way vision glass between two rooms, an arrangement that various team members had found useful for teaching in other settings.

In the absence of a trained medical psychiatric staff, the psychology and social work departments of the hospital had assumed the major responsibility for essential psychiatric decisions about patients, and whatever psychotherapy was done at Midwest was the province of the psychologists. Everyone at the hospital, from the Superintendent to the ward attendants—and including all of the clinical departments—shared the conviction at the time that the need with highest priority was for well-trained psychiatric specialists, preferably on a full-time basis. These same people also felt that if full-time psychiatrists were not available, the present doctors, if offered some on-the-spot teaching, were sufficiently interested in psychiatric problems to warrant an investment in their training. The top administrators observed that at least some of the doctors might, with such instruction, abandon their plans to "escape" from the hospital as soon as an Illinois medical license became available.

It may be useful at this point for the reader to be introduced individually, as the new team was, to the hospital's chief personnel. The following notes are taken from the coordinator's report to the team at the time of his reconnaissance visit.

Superintendent, Dr. Gordon

The Superintendent is ill with his second coronary occlusion at this time. He seems to be revered by everyone as a permissive but also firm leader and father-figure. He is the one who put through the open-door policy, even against the darkest warnings of his fiercely loyal chief nurse, who has been in state hospital service for thirty years. Apparently, the success of this program has increased everyone's conviction about the omniscience of their leader. His heart attack, however, seems to have shattered their fantasies of his omnipotence (in contrast to his omniscience), and the hospital personnel have become anxious about the future. Two of the top doctors promptly took jobs elsewhere. Routines are disrupted, and the personnel are looking around hopefully for new leadership. In one sense, this constitutes a danger for our team. If we entered the scene at this time, we might be seized upon irrationally as the new Messiahs. On the other hand, this disrupted state of affairs could work in our favor if we are able to use it wisely and temperately.

Acting Clinical Director, Dr. Burke

Dr. Burke comes from Poland. Acutely aware of his lack of training for his job, he rides his staff mercilessly; he mistrusts them and considers them lazy. When I asked him how the consultants could be most helpful to the staff, he replied that half days of consultation with problem cases and perhaps two hours of lectures might be ideal. When I asked what he meant by lectures, I found that what he had in mind were seminars in which the consultants would answer the doctors' questions. He anticipated difficulty with lectures, however, because he felt it would be impossible to get the doctors all together at one time.[1] They need training in basic psychiatry and neurology. He suggested that the consultants work in the acute diagnostic and treatment unit only, which is where he has assigned the two staff physicians whom he believes are interested in becoming psychiatrists.

Staff Physician, Dr. Samuels

Dr. Samuels also comes from Poland. He is forty-eight years old, and his English is only fair. He is one of the two doctors who, according to the Clinical Director, are interested in psychiatry, and for that reason he is assigned to the Admissions Building. He has been at Midwest since last year, working first on chronic wards, then being assigned to the intensive treatment building. He worked

---

[1] In retrospect, we see this statement as probably an early manifestation · of resistance to the project on the part of the hospital administration.

in mental hospitals in another country for three years, mainly with chronic cases. He has a state license, has not decided whether or not to become a psychiatrist, and feels he cannot afford to go elsewhere for residency training. Although he likes psychiatry, he needs more money and therefore may go into general practice in a small town. At this point he is undecided. When I asked him how this hospital compares with others he has worked in, he said it compares well. The chief problem is the lack of psychiatric specialists. Some of the doctors are a problem, he added; he considers himself such a problem in that he has had no real training in psychiatry and much of the time does not know what to do with his patients. How could the consultants help most, I asked. He suggested that we interview patients for the doctors and tell them what to do. He feels that he does not even know where to find good articles to read on subjects such as tranquilizers. I asked whether there is anything besides staffing patients that is needed and would help. He then suggested that the physicians need training in basic psychiatry—such basic matters as classification, diagnostic principles, and the like. The doctors can make general diagnostic classifications, but they never know the more detailed issues. They also know general treatment measures, but not specific details about treatment. They feel cut off from psychiatric centers, left to themselves professionally, and they need advice and guidance about what to study.

Staff Physician, Dr. Bolley

Dr. Bolley is forty-three years old, from Lithuania, does not have a state license, and speaks English well. He came to the hospital this year, works in the medical and surgical building taking care of emergencies. He believes the greatest need of the medical staff is for training in psychiatry. His own interest in psychiatry is not so deep, he said; he may go into private medical practice. He has a large family, however, and for that reason is tempted to stay in state hospital work. If he were receiving training in psychiatry, he would be more inclined to remain at the hospital. The greatest problem, he said, is so many geriatric patients. Some of the hospital buildings—the infirmary, for example—are crowded with patients and have very poor living conditions. He felt that something should be done for them. They don't even have cool water to drink. The infirmary has a concrete floor on which the old patients slip, fall, and break their hips. He believes that something could be done—that morally these patients deserve more, after all their years of paying taxes! Dr. Bolley obviously has much interest in and compassion for old people. We might keep this interest of his in mind for a possible clinical research project with geriatric patients.

Staff Physician, Dr. Bernards

Dr. Bernards is also from Lithuania, is sixty-nine years old, and has been at the hospital for four years. His English is fair. He is responsible for six open wards, all chronic, with a total of three hundred and fifty patients, half of whom are on industrial assignments. He believes the hospital is better now. Why? Because the doctors can use tranquilizing medicines more freely. In addition, they have more open wards and a higher discharge rate. The industrial service is also better organized now; patients have a chance to live at the hospital and get jobs in the community. There is more for patients to do in occupational, recreational, and industrial therapy. Does he plan to stay at the hospital? Yes. What did he do previously? General practice, emphasizing eye. He doubts whether he will ever return to private practice. What is needed most at the hospital? Full-time psychiatrists. He does not believe that consultants would be enough help, although they would be better than nothing—especially if they give consultations on new patients at the Admissions Building. What about chronic patients—could the consultants help with them? Yes, they need much help with them, too. "We are not psychiatrists; we don't know what to do with them." I asked for an example. "Well, a patient may refuse to work or do anything. I don't know what to do with him. He may say he would help or work only if we paid him." Will the patients talk to you? "Yes, a little." Do you ever sit down and try to talk with individual patients? "I haven't much time for that—but occasionally I do, and I can see them respond." Are you interested in having training in psychiatry? "Yes, definitely." You wouldn't be embarrassed to undertake training at your age? "No, training never stops."[2] He added, however, that he might find it difficult to do the necessary reading and studying during the evenings.

Staff Physician, Dr. Christy

Dr. Christy is forty-eight years old, from Greece, and his English is fair. He has been in this country for four years, at Midwest for one. He has four wards, all chronic, and

---

[2]Dr. Bernards, despite his age, proved to be one of the most flexible and receptive to new ideas.

he said that the amount of work depends upon the number of staff physicians. At one time they had twelve doctors, but now there are only ten. What are his plans? He wants to get a state medical license and practice general medicine. Has he any interest in psychiatry? He has become interested in psychiatry and can conceive of staying in this field. He might stay at the hospital for several more years until his English improves more. He has trouble understanding patients who do not speak clearly. Would he be interested in psychiatric training by the consultants? Yes, he would; even if he does not stay at the hospital, the training would be useful in general practice. What would be most helpful to him? "Basic training in psychiatry—what to read, which books. Also, clinical help with problem patients." For example? "I have a catatonic patient who has been here for twenty years. I cannot get her out of the catatonic depression, have tried all medications, but nothing helps." Will she talk to you? "Yes, but all she says is, 'let me go home.'" Has anyone tried to figure out why she acts that way, what is going on in her mind? "No, we have given her shock treatment, and it, like everything else, failed."

Staff Physician, Dr. Simon

Dr. Simon is thirty-three years old, was born in the United States but raised in the Philippines. His English is perfect. He has been at Midwest only three weeks. He is in charge of the Admissions Building part of the week, but also sees family-care and conditional-discharge patients in nearby clinics each Wednesday and at three nursing homes in the area. He had a residency in general practice and surgery in Chicago, heard about this hospital, and came here because he likes psychiatry. He would like to have a residency in psychiatry. He makes rounds every day, writes progress notes every third, seventh, and fourteenth day, and then again a month later. He gives shock treatment to only two patients. He has never had training in psychiatry and would be very interested in such training from the consultant team. He thinks that an hour lecture once a week would be enough. Otherwise, he would suggest consultations on patients for diagnosis and treatment. Each such consultation, he felt, counting the discussion time, would probably take two hours. What are the outstanding problems at the hospital? "We need to have psychiatrists come and help us decide what to do."

Chief Psychiatric Social Worker, Mrs. Deutsch

Mrs. Deutsch has a Master's degree in social work. She complained that the doctors often do not follow through on the recommendations of the Acting Clinical Director, so the social workers try to do the follow-up on his recommendations (electroshock, drugs, occupational therapy) particularly on the chronic wards. She reported rivalry between the doctors and psychologists at the Admissions Building because the psychologists know more about psychiatry than the doctors do. Social workers have unusual influence and even authority because they are in on and to some extent control the staff evaluation of patients. Doctors often hardly know the patients being staffed. Because the doctors are transferred so frequently from one set of wards to another, the social workers end up being the ones who know the patients and therefore making the decisions. Mrs. Deutsch feels certain that the social work staff would respect and accept the recommendations of the psychiatric consultants. There are eight, including herself, on the social work staff. All except herself became psychiatric social workers through experience at the hospital. How could a psychiatric social work consultant be used? She suggested that a PSW consultant could help them handle problems in their relationships with the doctors, could help them to be more objective, could offer training in casework, and also could help them improve their work with families.

Acting Chief Psychologist, Dr. Shore[3]

Dr. Shore has been at the hospital for three years. The psychology staff consists of four psychologists, two having Ph.D.'s, one an M.A., and another completing his Master's degree. They have no interns in their department. Dr. Shore would be chiefly interested in consultants for psychotherapy. The psychologists are the only ones who do psychotherapy at the hospital, both individual and group therapy. The department is fairly isolated because there is no one they can call on for consultation and help. They get diagnostic consultations on ward-management problems from the Acting Clinical Director, but he is not trained in psychiatry. Ward problems are so numerous that the psychotherapy program is not receiving the attention it needs. What about the nature and extent of diagnostic and therapeutic activities in the psychology department? Well, whereas previously they did psychological work-ups on all patients, they now limit themselves to patients who are

[3] Dr. Shore was replaced by Dr. Hoy only a few months after the project got under way.

referred to the psychology department. Dr. Shore is the one who selects patients for diagnostic staffing. He hopes to free more time for his staff to do intensive psychotherapy. He would like to see the doctors become more willing and able to take psychiatric responsibility. The psychologists feel secure about their place at the hospital, he said, so they would welcome consultants. I repeated the question about the nature and extent of therapeutic activities by the psychology department. He then indicated that they have two therapy groups going, and each psychologist has two or three individual therapy patients who are seen two or three times a week. One of the problems is that patients often do not remain at the hospital long enough for them to continue the therapy to completion, and the staff is not allowed to do out-patient therapy. When patients leave the hospital, they are referred to the local clinic in Illinois City, which has a social worker, psychologist, and a part-time psychiatrist. The psychology staff limits its services to the diagnostic and treatment building due to staff shortages. They do a great deal of testing, he said, and also have much staffing of patients to do—most of which is done by what he calls "desk staffing," i.e., without seeing the patient. Their preference for a psychology consultant would be one who is expert in group therapy.

Chief Nurse, Mrs. Ott

Mrs. Ott has worked at the hospital for thirty years, and has been Chief Nurse for seven. Her department has twenty-two registered nurses, twelve licensed practical nurses, and sixteen licensed aides (not from aide schools, however). The aides are directly under her supervision.

Only four of her nurses are psychiatrically trained; these four work principally in the Admissions Building, one being in charge of all somatic therapy. I asked about nursing problems and needs. She first emphasized the need for improved facilities. The Medical and Surgical Building is dilapidated; many of the buildings are old, making the work more difficult. Aides are being trained as rapidly as possible, and she is trying to expand the nursing staff. What could psychiatric consultants do to help the nurses? The consultants should hold clinics, classes, ward discussions about patients and their needs, newer principles of treatment, and diagnosis. It would also help if the consultants would make out definite programs of treatment plans for patients so that the nurses would know what principles and plans to follow. She envisages the nurses' being brought in on discussions about the individual patients' problems and how they could better contribute to the patients' care and management. She feels that the present group of doctors is unusually sincere and willing to be trained; she also believes that the doctors would tend to stay on at the hospital longer if given training. Such a training program would not be disruptive, she said. "The place is already so disrupted, what we need is for someone to come in and restore some balance and get some routines set up."

Director of Activity Therapy, Miss Cotton

Miss Cotton has been in state service for thirty years, at this hospital for nine. Her department consists of four sections. Occupational Therapy has a section head and twelve staff personnel. They concentrate principally on arts and crafts, but also undertake certain other activities. The range of abilities among their patients is wide; many are alert and able, some stuporous.

Then there is Recreational Therapy, which has its own section head and again about twelve R.T. staff personnel, plus some extra college student helpers in the summertime. The summer students are good help, and they get a lot out of the work, which they carry with them into whatever field they enter. The recreational section utilizes, for the most part, music, dances, shows, bingo, and sports. They take large numbers of patients to symphony concerts, the circus, the county fair. The patients were taken to a public swimming pool this summer. for the first time; they are screened by the doctors, and their pool time is restricted. Frequent picnics are arranged for them in local parks, the sites being chosen by the patients themselves. An important feature of all this is that recreational activities have spread into the community, and the community is accepting the patients increasingly well. The members of the symphony orchestra, for example, consider the patients a good audience. Occupational and recreational therapy are often integrated — that is, occupational therapy in the morning, recreational therapy in the afternoon. Recreational therapy is considered not merely amusement, but treatment. This section of the Activity Therapy Department is also responsible for the patient government (council) and patient newspaper. A bandmaster gives musical instruction to as many patients as possible. Several choirs have been organized, and there is a rhythm band for regressed patients.

A third section of this department is the library, which has a full-time librarian and an assistant. The library has ten thousand volumes for patients and a medical-psychiatric-psychological-etc. technical section. The librarian visits the wards to determine what reading would be best for individual patients. The library receives about fifteen local daily newspapers so that patients from different communities can keep in touch with home. It also conducts classes for patients with language problems or other difficulties in communication.

Finally, there is Industrial Therapy, which is much like occupational therapy in its basic theory, but with abler patients. The hospital could not run without the patients who have industrial assignments: laundry, farm, lawn detail, etc. — approximately fifty different classifications of jobs. What are the main problems? The time problem of being unable to give patients the individual attention they need. The rehabilitation counselor works closely with the Director of Activity Therapy, having an office on the same floor. Their collaboration is helpful and necessary; it puts more pressure on patients to perform at the level expected of them in preparation for returning home. Is there any way psychiatric consultants could help? Yes, several ways. The staff physicians do not have time to come to the work areas. The activity therapists could use help in evaluating their programs of occupational, recreational, and industrial therapy. "We need to evaluate what we are doing. We do what we do largely by feel, a pragmatic approach. Are we going in the right direction? What criteria do we have for deciding? At Menninger's, they can tell you *why* they put a woman to scrubbing. Why does one patient respond and another not?" Does the activity therapy staff receive any training in basic psychiatric and psychopathologic theory? "Another state hospital has a school that gives a ten-week course in basic theory. We depend on them for such training."

The energetic and enthusiastic spirit of the Activity Therapy staff was in sharp contrast to the discouraged attitudes of the doctors and nurses. This initial impression was borne out by later experience and led to a special training project, conducted by one of the psychiatric consultants with the Activity Therapy staff.

The foregoing observations illustrate the importance of the manpower problem in large mental hospitals, especially the potentiality for improvement in this area. Numbers, here, were less significant than skill. The Activity Therapy Department had an excellent leader with the capacity for transmitting her enthusiasm and ideas to her staff. Admittedly, she had the most capable and trainable staff members to work with. It was for these reasons that, toward the end of the present project, the consultant team recommended to the Department of Health, Education and Welfare that if Domestic Service Corps workers were utilized in mental hospitals, they be assigned to the Activity Therapy Departments for their training and supervision.

The doctors and other personnel interviewed by the coordinator on his first visit were representative, of course, of a larger professional staff. In all, Midwest State Hospital at the beginning of the consultant team project had, in addition to its ten doctors, four psychologists, nine social workers, twelve nurses, sixteen trained aides, twenty-six occupational and recreational therapists, two librarians, and a Protestant and a Catholic chaplain. One measure of the problems inherent in shifting the focus of such a hospital from a custodial to a therapeutic one lies in these figures. Responsibility for the care of eighteen hundred patients rested with just eighty-one persons of greatly varied training and experience: the ratio of doctors to patients was about one to two hundred.

And, compared with some state hospitals, Midwest could be considered relatively *well* staffed.

Although preliminary interviews were not held with every member of the Midwest staff, some general observations could be made from the discussions that did take place. For one thing, the hospital physicians had no feeling of group cohesiveness—and this, in spite of a common background of escape from some painful situation in their homelands and a common situation of stress in their present jobs. The "group" was in actuality an assortment of individuals among whom cliques sprang up all too easily.

Furthermore, it seemed evident that none of the doctors really expected or hoped that he could, through any consulting program, ever attain professional autonomy as a psychiatrist. Instead, the doctors seemed to regard themselves as purveyors of orders from the consultant team, adopting a position of deferential submission to the "authority" from outside. This attitude may, in part, have reflected the monolithic administrative structure of Midwest State Hospital; it may also have had its roots in the rather authoritarian styles of living to which the physicians had always been accustomed.

The consultant team shared the view of many educators that a successful teaching-learning experience is characterized by teacher and learner striving for the same goals. It was therefore apparent that ways would have to be devised, or improvised, to promote a more hopeful orientation among the physicians and to encourage their latent strivings toward professional autonomy in a new specialty. At the same time, the consultant team would have to make a constant effort to resist any temptation to exercise authority in a noneducational way.

Faced with an institution of the size and complexity of Midwest State Hospital, the members of the new consultant team needed more than their city-bred professional skills and knowledge. Perhaps above all they—and their hospital colleagues—needed optimism, energy, and a willingness to learn from each other. How the hospital staff and the consultant team learned from each other is the subject of the following chapters.

CHAPTER THREE

The Project in Progress

The First Visits

WITHIN THREE MONTHS of the submission and approval of the proposal to organize a consultant team, the team was recruited, Midwest State Hospital was selected, and the consultants had made an initial joint visit to the hospital.

By the end of the following month, all the consultants had spent at least one Friday at Midwest. Slowly, the new environment evolved into a real place with real people. It soon became apparent that each consultant had preformed expectations about the level of sophistication of the "students" and the teaching approach to be used, expectations that later underwent considerable revision. For example, the team was aware that all of the doctors were foreign-born and none trained in psychiatry, but appreciated the implications of these facts only with experience. In their first reports, the psychiatric consultants were uniformly impressed with the enthusiasm and liveliness of the medical staff, but they became increasingly dismayed by the doctors' poor preparation for psychiatric work. These men, who were highly competent in their original medical specialties, were downright afraid of approaching psychiatric patients. Clearly, they had been concentrating on the medical problems of their patients, some maintaining friendly, fatherly relationships with the patients, others appearing in their wards only briefly, and avoiding personal contacts. The doctors' natural inclination to think in terms of disease entities, of diagnosing and categorizing patients, took the form of questions focused on clarifying terminology—the differences between psychoses and neuroses, between ego and personality, between illusion, delusion, and hallucination. The neurological consultant was slightly more impressed with the doctors' level of knowledge than his psychiatric colleagues were. In the neurological field, the staff doctors were on firmer ground and could display and utilize their previous training.

The consultants also became concerned about a punitive attitude toward patients who did not conform. One consultant commented, "They all need to learn a more tender approach," and another said, "Another group attitude, which we are going to have to work with by demonstration, is a rather prevalent one of criticism toward the patient's neurotic behavior. It is as though they were afraid that the patient was going to put something over on them, a feeling exemplified in the social workers' questioning and in the comments of some of the doctors: 'The patient is institution-trained'; 'He knows how to get around the staff.' "

The consultants gradually learned to differentiate among the doctors. A few seemed to have a natural aptitude for psychiatric work, while others seemed bored and lethargic, and at least one expressed fear at the prospect of undertaking individual psychiatric interviews. A consultant said, "I am sure they are not uniformly interested in the wares we peddle . . . my feeling is that they are all interested in learning something about psychiatry and neurology, even though they may not make it a career. . . . A few, I am sure, will stay on for one reason or another."

Miss Jacob discovered that the Social Service staff was preoccupied primarily with intake and discharge activities and had little other contact with the patients. There was an active Family Care program, with much attention devoted to seeking out appropriate patients and preparing them for transfer to Family Care. Dr. Stock found that the psychologists were busy in the community outside the hospital, giving lectures to various local organizations. Generally, the consultants were disappointed with the performance of both psychologists and social workers, especially during the morning case conferences when the members of those disciplines who had been involved with the patient were present and reported their findings. The psychologist at these conferences often was speculative, relying more heavily on interview data than data from his diagnostic testing. The personal histories presented by the social workers were sometimes sketchy and poorly organized. In their therapeutic work with patients, the psychologists were inclined to set unrealistic goals; they seemed to expect a major reconstruction of personality, and were disappointed and discouraged when this failed to occur.

The consultants also discovered how poor communication was among hospital personnel. So unaccustomed were members of the staff to discussing their activities and their patients, that in many instances several persons working with the same patient failed to keep in touch with each other and, in consequence, worked at cross purposes. In addition, there were clouds on the horizon with respect to the hospital administration. At first, the welcome had been warm and the top administration seemed to feel honored at having been selected for the consultant team project. Within weeks, however, this positive attitude had been sounded and was proving rather shallow. The coordinator of the project reported on an early interview with the Superintendent:

> My reason for spending some time with Dr. Gordon was primarily to get better acquainted with him and, if possible, to build up a relationship of trust and partnership between us. That may not be easy to do, since he has a tendency to be rather hale and hearty about everything, rather than wanting to tackle some of the difficult problems we face. I asked him to let me know about any indications of dissatisfaction with our program, but he assured me magnanimously that he has heard nothing but praise.

At this time, without the consultant's team's knowledge Dr. Gordon was making arrangements for the staff physicians to attend a course in psychology at a local college, a move he considered his prerogative, regardless of the consultant team's view that additional training should not be undertaken, or undertaken only if it fitted into the existing program.

That the doctors were foreign born and psychiatrically naïve and the psychologists and social workers were native born and trained created another uncomfortable area. Both groups were dealing with this awkwardness by withdrawing from one another. The consultant team, without realizing it at the time, interfered with this pattern of isolation by bringing personnel together for the diagnostic conferences. The first hint of possible trouble was the glee expressed by some doctors when a psychologist or social worker was challenged by a consultant. It took time for the consultants to realize that some of the most irritating hospital events, such as the personnel's leaving the job on long lunch breaks or accepting outside speaking engagements, were in fact understandable reactions to a situation filled with stress.

During these early weeks, in spite of disappointments, the consultants found that their morale remained high and their interest constantly engaged. But a day at the hospital was exhausting for every member of the team. Several of them reported feeling as tired as after a week of work in their usual settings. This feeling of exhaustion was probably related to an acute awareness of the needs of the patients and staff, and a parallel frustration at not being able to do more, more quickly. As each consultant settled down to concentrating his efforts on what could be done in the time available, the feeling of exhaustion dropped away.

After the first visit or two, all the consultants found themselves modifying their teaching approaches. These modifications ranged from choosing words carefully for the benefit of doctors whose English was poor, to changing the day's schedule in order to respond to some need or interest of the group. One consultant, for example, canceled his individual conferences in order to discuss in a seminar the doctors' many questions about a patient presented at the morning conference. Toward the end of the first month, the team agreed that the doctors needed direct help in history-taking, and it was decided that one of the team would prepare a guide. We also decided to postpone working with the doctors on ward milieu problems until they were better grounded in basic psychiatry.

Digging In

Following the initial visits, came a digging-in period for both the consultants and the hospital personnel. As the two groups began to know each other better, the trip reports began to reflect a greater appreciation of the hospital as a community and an alertness to the mutual impact of team and hospital.

The first observable impact of the teaching was in the doctors' attitude toward patients and fellow staff members, a change that seemed to result from identification with the consultants. One of the doctors told a consultant that he now paid closer attention to the social history because he noticed that the consultants always did so. Another commented that, since observing that the consultants always began an interview with what the patient wanted to talk about, he was trying that technique. About midway in the first year of the project, a team member reported that "staff are noticeably less suspicious and hostile toward patients—that is, they are more secure."

But even as the consultants reported progress in learning, so they noted new resistances to training. Having observed that the physicians needed such extensive help in their actual clinical contacts with patients, the consultants began to press them to take on a few patients in psychotherapy, under supervision. One of the consultants noted the resistance to such suggestions during a conference with the doctors on psychotherapy.

Dr. Samuels said that he thought psychotherapy was a "very drastic treatment" and frankly admitted he was frightened. He felt he might get the patient's confidence, but what then? Did he have a right to "force" psychotherapy on a patient who did not want it? Also, he was concerned about his authoritative position as a physician — couldn't he harm the patient in some way? Dr. Burke raised a very interesting question regarding the effect of the therapist's neurosis on the therapy. . . . I think there is a good deal of concern, too, in the "Latin Block" about moral attitudes. I think they need a good deal of help as a group with the fears of doing irreparable damage to the patient through psychotherapy. Dr. Simon was concerned about how to handle dependency, and was it a good thing or a bad thing? Someone wanted to know how you could tell when the therapy was completed.

A few doctors were willing, in spite of their fears, to undertake psychotherapy with patients, and, with them, the individual consultant conferences were devoted to case supervision. As more doctors began to conduct therapeutic interviewing with patients, regular supervision was established by a preceptor system, which provided for each psychiatric consultant to supervise four doc-doctors, so that a continuing relationship could be maintained. In addition to their supervisory sessions, the doctors were encouraged to telephone the consultants long distance when special problems or emergencies arose.

From the beginning, the doctors were relatively receptive to the teaching of neurology, doubtless because the contents and concepts of neurology, being more directly related to medicine, were more familiar to them. The patient population provided examples of many neurological diseases, and the frequent coincidence of psychiatric disorders allowed opportunities for correlations of the disciplines. Thus, the inclusion of neurology in the curriculum served the double purpose of engaging the doctors in a familiar medical discipline while simultaneously imparting knowledge in organic psychiatry and neurology.

As they came to know the staff better, the consultants became concerned about poor communication within the hospital. Social workers, for example, visited relatives of patients without any communication with the patients' ward physicians. The new Chief Psychologist, Dr. Hoy, complained to one of the consultants that Dr. Simon seldom referred patients for psychological testing. Confronted with this remark, Dr. Simon said he did not refer patients because he knew the psychologists were overworked. As the consultant observed, "Simon's sending few patients for psychological testing turns out to be essentially an act of love, but lack of communication between Hoy and Simon results in her taking his behavior to be hostile." At about the same time, Dr. Hoy complained about the manner in which one of the doctors conducted intake staffings. She said that he asked for social service reports, but that anyone else who wanted to comment about the patient had to fight for time. He saw the patient for about a minute, then, with no discussion at all, dictated a diagnostic summary and treatment recommendations, with the rest of the staff as audience. Dr. Hoy commented that, by this time, if one disagreed with the diagnosis, it seemed impossible to say so.

There were even instances of a patient's being discharged by a ward physician without any conference with the psychologist conducting therapy with the patient. On the reverse side of the coin, the ward physician sometimes did not even know the patient was receiving psychotherapy from a psychologist. The consultants could and did have some impact on this problem of communication, largely by showing what a high value they placed on interdepartmental discussion and collaboration by the staff. One consultant, while talking to a doctor about one of his patients, asked if he had read the nurse's notes. He had not. Whereupon they then did just that and talked to the nurses as well, "who seemed a bit baffled, but also pleased to be asked about a patient's behavior on the ward."

At the staff's suggestion, an Education Committee was organized for the purpose of coordinating all the training activities within the hospital. This committee included the Clinical Director and the various Department Heads; the coordinator of the Consultant Team was invited to attend the monthly meetings. A psychiatric consultant began to work with an interdisciplinary staff group on a double-blind drug study; another psychiatric consultant agreed to work with an alcoholic project initiated by Dr. Hoy, the Chief Psychologist. The Education Committee also eased the communication problem by deciding that if a matter concerning follow-up came to the attention of a social worker or psychologist connected with a particular case, they would discuss the problem with the patient's doctor, who, in turn, would discuss it with the consultant if necessary. If a joint conference of doctor-psychologist-social worker with the consultant seemed indicated, part of that doctor's individual conference time might be scheduled for such a discussion. In that case, the doctor's individual conference time would be lengthened so that he would not have to sacrifice his time alone with the consultant. While such developments helped, it was many months before barriers began to break down and the staff members voluntarily sought one another out to talk about particular patients.

One of the problems besetting Midwest was the constant changes in personnel. During the first year, one new doctor arrived and two left; three new psychologists, one of them the Chief Psychologist, were added to the staff, as was one social worker. During the second year further important changes occurred. Five new doctors arrived and had to be integrated into the program. Dr. Simon became Acting Clinical Director, replacing Dr. Burke, who left to undertake residency training in psychiatry. One ward physician resigned during the summer between the first and second years, and Dr. Hoy, the Chief Psychologist, left in the spring of the second year. The latter was an especially important loss, both because she had been very capable and because she could not be replaced immediately.

These changes caused a noticeable dip in morale. When the two doctors resigned toward the end of the first year, one of the other doctors told a consultant that he was thinking about leaving in a few months and that three other doctors might also leave. This ward physician had come to work at the hospital because he had no money and needed a job and shelter for his family. When the consultant team came along, he decided to stay. But with two doctors now gone, he was afraid that the hospital would again — as it had the year before — be reduced to four or five doctors. He had already had to take on some additional chronic wards.

Rather quickly, the consultants learned that these staff changes, as well as a variety of other crises, were recurring, to-be-expected features of the state hospital. We began to see the hospital itself as a durable institution which would always deal somehow with the problems experienced and created by its staff and consultants. The consultants met these crises as philosophically as they could. One reported:

> Dr. Reese told me that the whole hospital was upset, and he wanted me to know it was because the State has stopped the food allowance without making a compensatory increase in pay. For those with large families, this means in effect a salary reduction of two hundred dollars a month or more. Dr. Reese had been somewhat on the fence about staying around, feeling that always before he had been treated fairly, but now has no alternative to leaving as soon as he possibly can. He is going to take the state board exams soon. It all sounds as if they are trying to freeze out the state hospitals, but I found myself reflecting that for many years to come there is going to be a Midwest State Hospital, whether or not they have either staff or consultant team. The hospital itself is permanent.

Another consultant:

> While I do not consider these storms to be harmless, I have become resigned to the inevitability of this periodic emotional violence, particularly between the administrators and the ward physicians. I have grown to feel that since there is nothing that one seems able to do to prevent these disturbances, all we can do is

learn to be prepared for them and go right on working in and around them when they occur.

Still another consultant, concerning another kind of recurrent crisis:

> I took a train on Thursday evening. It was five and a half hours late, arriving at 6:30 A.M. The steam line was broken, so there was no heat on the train. When I got off this refrigerator car, it was too late to check into the hotel. For the return trip, there was a two and a half hour delay until the plane took off. When I phoned my wife to tell her that the plane would be delayed, I asked her to have me locked up if she ever saw me setting out for this place again.

An encouraging feature of the first year was the development of interdisciplinary projects. The team was gratified to find that those staff members who had originally expressed an interest in a particular area were eager to follow up on it. A wide variety of projects were accordingly developed, with a psychiatric consultant working with Dr. Bolley and the hospital administration in developing an experimental geriatric program, and the psychology consultant with Dr. Bernards and several of his aides in developing a milieu program for one of his female wards. This program faltered temporarily when none of the other doctors proved interested in it, but it revived later on. In addition, a Volunteers Project was established, as well as the Alcoholic Project, which survived the departure of Dr. Hoy, its guiding spirit. A Psychopharmacology Project also got under way; this was subsequently given special financial support by the State.

Stimulated by their concern about the anxiety

aroused in patients upon their initial admission to a mental hospital ward, the psychiatric social work and psychology staffs collaborated in the development of a New-Patient Orientation Project. The psychology and psychiatric social work consultants served as advisers to the project, which provided that patients newly admitted to the hospital be invited and encouraged to attend new-patient meetings dealing specifically with problems of initial adjustment.

Finally, there was a Journal Club, formed by the Superintendent and the Clinical Director. This club included staff members from the Medical, Psychology, and Psychiatric Social Work Departments, who met regularly to discuss selected articles from the literature of those fields.

Conflict continued to arise from time to time between the consultant team and the hospital administration regarding their areas of function and jurisdiction. It was assumed on both sides that a boundary could and should be drawn, but in practice that boundary proved to be elusive. The Superintendent or Clinical Director might regard a decision made by the consultants—one the consultants considered as part of the teaching program—as an invasion of their prerogatives as administrators. Similarly, the team felt that some of the decisions made by the hospital administration unduly restricted the teaching program. For instance, when the consultants urged the doctors to conduct supervised psychotherapy of individual patients as part of the training program, the Superintendent blocked this program for several months by not making individual interviewing rooms available to the medical staff. At that time the ward physicians were not permitted to have individual offices on or near their wards, but were required to do any office work at the administration building, where each of the doctors had a desk in the same large room and where the Superintendent and Clinical Director could "keep an eye on them." In this instance, the Consultant Team resorted to bypassing the Superintendent's passive resistance by encouraging the ward physicians to find secluded corners of their wards — this often turned out to be the ward linen closet — for individual interviews with patients.

The team's feeling about the hospital administration during the first year was summarized by the coordinator: "So far, I have been unable to make much progress in establishing a real working partnership with Dr. Gordon. I continue to have the feeling that we are working in his hospital, but that somehow we are not working *with* him." Sometimes, these conflicts could be resolved by talking them over with the hospital administration, but it proved impossible to arrive at general policies that would prevent other problems from arising. The assumption that a clear boundary could be drawn between consultation and administration was probably incorrect, since, in fact, a large number of decisions involved both groups, and no procedure was ever developed for distinguishing clearly between them. This conflict was finally reduced, although never entirely resolved, quite by chance, with the arrival, in the third year of the project, of a new Superintendent whose ideas were more congruent with those of the team.[1]

[1] In the second state hospital project, this issue was dealt with more satisfactorily through a steering committee composed of the hospital's top administration, the coordinator of the consultant team, and heads of the various departments at the hospital. Any projected change in the teaching program, arising from any source, was discussed by this committee, and a decision made. One thing learned from the Midwest experience is that the impact of a consultant team on a hospital is certain to be jarring and that some mechanism has to be provided for dealing with the ensuing problems and tensions.

Another question having to do with boundaries—"When do or should consultation and supervision become therapy?"—presented little difficulty. The team was careful not to become therapists to staff members, but it was often both appropriate and necessary to deal with emotional resistance to learning. The single case of a rather serious personality problem was helped to enter private psychotherapy.

Anxieties or resentments stirred up by the consultant program sometimes came to the attention of the team only indirectly. As just one of several examples, a team member heard that the Chief Nurse had spoken resentfully about the geriatric project, which was still in an embryonic stage. The team coordinator promptly sought out the Chief Nurse and told her that it had come to his attention that she was not happy about some of the plans being made about the geriatric project and hoped she would be completely frank with him about this. She was. She blew up in a first-class catharsis about having been told to provide extra nurses for this project when she had only twenty-two nurses for the whole hospital. He waited until the abreaction died down and then told her that we were opposed to having other parts of the hospital stripped of nurses for the sake of this one small project. He assured her that we would straighten this out with Dr. Gordon and urged her to contact him directly in the future whenever problems of this kind arose. She promised to do so.

Fluctuations in staff attitudes toward the consultant team were constantly apparent. One consultant wrote, "I wonder for how many of the doctors the weekly visit of the consultant offers a respite from the tedium of their work and represents a kind of play or something to fill the time." According to another, "The doctors would hate to see us leave because we are helpful to them; but, on the other hand, I think they resent us currently because they look upon us as one more demand on their time and energies." And a third reported that, "The Clinical Director has said that Midwest now has a better program for the doctors than [Hospital X], which has always been considered the jewel of the rural hospital system."

In any event, it became clear that, as the team began to threaten some of the established procedures at the hospital, the administration became less enthusiastic. Variations in morale among particular personnel seemed very much related to whether the individual felt the master of, or overwhelmed by, the new demands being made upon him. Morale improved when therapeutic results became evident, as demonstrated by a hospital social worker who talked with pleasure and surprise about the fact that all patients studied by the con: ltant team seemed to have shown considerable improvement or at least significant change in some way. The consultant discussed with her the fact that this probably had to do both with a better understanding of the case and with the interest focused on these particular patients.

As the special projects were introduced and set into action, staff morale improved perceptibly, for these projects originated in response to special interests of staff members and to follow them through gave a much needed lift to their self-esteem. The coordinator reported that "Dr. Bolley told me he has come to feel very happy about having the assignment to the geriatric project. He indicated that he had pretty much decided to remain at Midwest indefinitely."

By the end of the first year, a great deal had been altered at the hospital and in the teaching program. The curriculum had been modified, special projects had started, and new working relationships were established. Perhaps the most notable single feature of the teaching program was flexibility and change; Fridays at Midwest were never routine or static. The program was full of difficulties, satisfactions, frustrations, delights, and exasperations.

Forging Ahead

When it came time to plan for the second year of the project, the team coordinator met with the hospital doctors in order to get their views and suggestions. They reiterated their pleas for more practical help with patients and less stress on theoretical subjects. The consultants, although unwilling to abandon their efforts to teach theory, agreed to modify the program in order to provide more practical help by lengthening the individual conferences so that each doctor was seen for a full hour, and by substituting Grand Rounds for the morning Diagnostic Conference. The latter change would make it possible to deal with patients in their own ward settings under circumstances more closely approximating those faced daily by the staff. The importance of the new projects was recognized, and regular meeting times were scheduled for these during the afternoons. The neurological, social service, and psychological consultants developed plans within their own departments.

The consultants were now regularly receiving new demands for service and, in response, slowly expanded their teaching efforts to include other hospital departments.

A request from the Activity Therapy Department resulted, early in the second year, in a new series of seminars conducted by one of the psychiatrists of the Chicago Team. At about the same time, the Protestant Chaplain requested supervision; the team's psychiatric social work consultant began meeting with him regularly. The social workers began meeting with groups of patients, in response to which the psychology consultant began a series of meetings with them concerning new patients. The hospital staff seemed eager to make as much use of the team as possible, and it became the usual thing for one or more staff members to ride out to the airport with the consultants, using that time for further discussion about a patient or a project. Some of the team members also began to schedule informal meetings on Thursday evenings, when they arrived from Chicago. When some of them began to feel overburdened, the team agreed that such extra commitments would be an individual matter, to be determined by each consultant's inclination and energy.

The consultants' notes continued to report both progress and problems on the part of the doctors and other staff members. One recurring problem was that the cultural and religious backgrounds of some staff members interfered with their maintaining a therapeutic attitude about human behavior and misbehavior. An example: "His religious morality showed up in an unpsychiatric light with a patient who is a manic-depressive man with two previous hospitalizations.... The patient had run off from his wife and family and lived with another woman. While describing this, the doctor said in a tone of distaste that, 'He even had sexual relations before marriage.... He doesn't even feel guilty about this.' "

There were also repeated instances of inappropriate punitive attitudes toward patients and lack of cooperation among the various departmental staffs. The social workers sometimes tended to identify with a patient's relatives, and the psychologists with the patient, whereupon the two groups declared war on each other and were quite unable to work cooperatively on the problem confronting both of them.

There were also indications of foot-dragging. A psychiatric consultant described an afternoon seminar with the doctors:

> Although I had made an explicit assignment in Louis Linn's *Handbook*, no one had read it. The excuse was that there was only one copy in the library. "Did anyone use that one copy?" Dead silence. So I carefully wrote the name of the author and the title on the board, and spelled out chapter and verse. I asked for a volunteer to report next time, and Dr. Jenny raised her hand. Then I lent her my copy. The meeting became more or less a bull session, which they are getting extremely good at using defensively.

But there was also progress, as evidenced by the following excerpts from trip reports:

> The conferences with my perceptees were uneventful, except to note continuing progress. Polonsky has begun on his own to interview and study certain alcoholics and their personality structures and has discussed with me a great many of his observations. I encouraged him and felt that this was evidence that he was getting interested and was not afraid to get his feet wet in the interpersonal situation. . . . Together with this report is enclosed a case history that Dr.

Jenny did, which I feel is in almost every respect an outstanding example of her progress in one year's time. I brought this up to the entire staff at the case conference and suggested to Dr. Simon that he circularize it, especially among the new doctors, as an example of a succinct and valuable case history.

Dr. Phillips' interest in occupational therapy is beginning to pay off. A couple of patients in his ward who formerly sat around all day are now making good progress in "coming back to life" as a result of his carefully thought out activities therapy programs.

Another example of Phillips' conscientiousness is recording of the case conferences and then going over the tapes in the evening, to improve both his understanding of the conference and his English.

Communication continued to be a problem, but there were indications of a happier trend. The coordinator reported that the Education Committee:

was unanimous in its wish to give information about projects to those not involved. I asked if a project could become known to everybody just by casual discussion, and their answers gave me the impression that there isn't such sharing of ideas and shop talk amongst themselves at the hospital. I told them I though that was too bad, and we discussed the possibility of an all-day or two-day institute at the hospital, perhaps once a year, in which reports would be presented on the various projects. . . .

Nearly a year later, it was reported that one of the hospital psychologists mentioned something that was especially good to hear— that since the consultant team has been working at the hospital, for the first time the psychologists find themselves able to discuss patients with the doctors in psychological terms. He said that discussions in dynamic psychological terms are frequent nowadays between the doctors, psychologists, and psychiatric social workers.

Jurisdictional disputes of the kind already described continued to arise between the consultant team and the hospital administration. But along with these current conflicts came moments of good feeling and sympathy. The team learned to present major plans to Dr. Gordon before their implementation; both the revised curriculum for the second year, and the first-year progress report were first reviewed by him. One of the consultants was also able to help Dr. Gordon with a difficult personnel problem; and when Gordon was attacked by several veterans' organizations for considering using the hospital's farm (previously devoted to veterans) for an adolescent unit, the sympathies of the team were with the Superintendent.

Perhaps the most emphatic vote of confidence in the consultants came during the second year when some of the hospital buildings were renamed. In a gesture unique among state institutions, Midwest dedicated and renamed one of its buildings in honor of Sigmund Freud, the founder of psychoanalysis. The consultant-team coordinator gave the dedication speech at the unveiling of a plaque on the building, and the consultant team presented the hospital with a portrait of Freud.

Late in the second year of the project Dr. Gordon died suddenly of a heart attack. Within a week, Dr. Burton Fisher, who had formerly been a staff member of another Illinois state hospital, arrived to take over the job of

Superintendent. The coordinator attended Dr. Gordon's funeral as the representative of the consultant team, and, just two days after the funeral, two other consultants made the next regularly scheduled visit to the hospital. Both observed a mood of lethargy and depression among the staff, evidently a reaction to Dr. Gordon's death. At the same time, the staff began to mythologize the new Superintendent idealistically, describing, for example, his "phenomenal memory." The team doubted whether Dr. Fisher, no matter how good he was, would be able to live up to the expectations the staff had of him.

The new Superintendent made an excellent impression on the consultant team; one of the psychiatric consultants observed:

> Dr. Fisher indicated that he agrees with our plan to break the hospital down into three, smaller independent units. He also wants to establish an out-patient department, increase personnel, etc. I think you will agree that he thinks very much as we do about the improvements needed at the hospital and how to bring them about.

The plan referred to, the Unit Team system, was instituted three months after Dr. Fisher's arrival. This system, which the consultant team had been thinking about for many months, divided the hospital into three smaller units, each staffed by its own interdisciplinary clinical team; and the patients admitted to a particular unit remained under the care of the same team throughout their hospitalization. Because each unit had its own admitting wards, chronic wards, infirmary beds, and out-patient services, patients progressed through the various services of the unit to which they had been admitted, but were never "handed around," as had happened formerly, to different staff personnel.

As the new unit system got underway, the consultant team was reorganized so that each psychiatric consultant worked with a particular unit, attending its staff meetings and functioning as preceptor to the doctors of that unit. After much turmoil, the hospital staff gradually found ways to cope with the new system and to make it work. Once they became committed to the unit system, no one thought of returning to the old arrangement.

The new unit teams almost immediately increased both the need and opportunity for communication among the staff. The psychology consultant reported: "Over-all, the most striking thing is the fact that it is beginning to be important to people to know and understand one another. In both the Psychology and Social Service staffs I found people sharing views about what their co-team members were really like. Notes were compared, especially, about the three Unit Chiefs, what could be expected from them, how they must be dealt with, etc."

But fresh problems also arose as a result of the new system. The psychology consultant reported that one of the social workers, Miss Rose, had instituted group therapy with some chronic ward women patients and, as a result, ". . . some of the doctors on the others units are feeling a little envious and putting pressure on the social workers in their own units to do the things Miss Rose is doing. She then gets repercussions from this."

Since the new Unit Chiefs had to assume more responsibility for diagnosis and therapeutic planning for patients, they began requesting more psychological tests; as a result, the psychologists soon found themselves buried under an avalanche of referrals. This crisis began to be resolved when the psychologists shared the problem with their unit teams and took a more active part in deciding whether testing was required for a particular patient.

Through the unit-team system, the consultants automatically became involved with a much wider range of hospital staff and personnel, including all those who attended intake and evaluation conferences of each unit: nurses, activity therapists, and aides, as well as doctors, social workers, and psychologists.

While much of the energy of both the consultant team and the hospital staff was devoted to the new unit teams, the usual group seminars and individual conferences continued. With the innovations in teaching, the teachers noted further progress in learning. A psychiatric consultant, reporting on some joint supervision with two staff doctors, said: "It is my impression that this joint supervision is useful: the discussion is lively, and the competition in showing what they know proves advantageous." In a subsequent report, he added:

> My meeting with the nurses was, I believe, one of the best I have had with them so far. When I came into the room, one of them asked me, "What did you tell Alice J. to do?" She went on to say that the patient had told her that I said she should cry any time she wants to. This was the springboard for discussing this patient and the process of mourning. We discussed how the nurse could be a therapeutic factor in fostering the working through of mourning.

The psychology consultant reported a new joint seminar on group therapy with the psychology and social work staffs:

We discussed the talkative patient; the patient who monopolizes; feelings that get aroused in the therapists when they discover that the patients can sometimes help one another more than the professionals can; problems that arise when patients assume that the group is to be conducted like a classroom; what to do when two or three conversations go on at once; and so forth.

Throughout the discussion I was very impressed, as usual, with the way Miss Rose has taken to this activity. Her own good sense and sensitivity carry her through, and she's clearly operating in her groups with great effectiveness and is also very useful to the two younger, less experienced social workers on her team.

Looking Ahead

From the beginning the consultant project was seen as a time-limited, three-year program, and from the beginning it was hoped that a local team of consultants could be organized to continue the work. Accordingly, during the second year, feelers were put out to which four psychiatrists and one neurosurgeon responded. With these as a nucleus, the Illinois-City consultant team[2] was formed during the summer between the second and third years of the project. In the ensuing several months, each of the new consultants accompanied one of the Chicagoans on his hospital visits. Early in the third year of the project, the consultants realized that the I-C team was ready and eager to work independently. It was agreed that the transition period should not be too extended and that the

[2]Chapter 8 describes the Illinois City consultant team in further detail.

I-C team should become more active and the Chicago team less active after the middle of the third year. During this time, the Chicagoans became participant observers, offering their help to the I-C consultants, but leaving the conduct of the conferences and the supervision in the hands of the new team. At the end of the third year, the Chicago team maintained contact with the I-C team through the Chicago-team coordinator, who received copies of the I-C trip reports, and also met occasionally with the I-C team coordinator and consultants.

Leaving the hospital was difficult for the Chicago consultant team, for it meant giving up and ceding to others relationships and programs that had developed considerable meaning for each member of the team. Mingled with relief at the prospect of more relaxation and less pressure was some concern that the I-C team might change — or even damage — the program. By the end of the third year, however, these worries had abated, and the consultants felt ready to leave, confident in the enthusiasm and competence of the I-C team, pleased that some contact would be retained with the hospital, involved in the task of writing the story about the three years at Midwest, and planning for a second consultant team project at an even larger and more isolated state hospital in Illinois.

CHAPTER FOUR

Toward Team Functioning

MOST OF THE CONSULTANTS' ACCOMPLISHMENTS at Midwest resulted from group action, from the implementation of the ideas of individuals by teams of professional workers. With the exception of the original plan for a coordinated group of consultants, however, the development of teams was unpremeditated rather than a predetermined plan. Teams arose out of necessity as it became clear that more could be accomplished in concert than in isolation.

There were a few antecedents of team functioning at the hospital prior to our arrival there. For the most part, however, these had to do with collaborative efforts between the hospital and the outside community: a radio program on prevention of mental illness, frequent speeches and panel discussions throughout the area, and other activities involving the relationship of the hospital to the "nonhospital." Within the institution, there were a few such attempts at working together. Among these were occasional general staff meetings, the hospital newspaper (which brought together, on paper at least, information about the different departments), annual picnics, award ceremonies of various kinds, and, in scattered instances, some private collaboration between the Vocational Rehabilitation Counselor and the Director of the Activity Therapy Department. The relatively new open-door policy may also have stimulated greater "openness" between departments, as well as some banding together by the staff out of anxiety lest "the patients get out."

But all of these examples of interdepartmental communication were unrelated to the primary function of the hospital: patient care. Within that area, the staff was widely separated and the idea of collaborative planning for patients was a thing unknown. Even on social occasions, the staff members grouped themselves into departmental clusters—a tendency so far-reaching that members of different disciplines often did not know one another by name.

The evolution toward team functioning probably resulted from the example and the efforts of the consultant team. The example was constant: throughout the years at Midwest, the staff could observe the consultants working together effectively and *by choice*. Efforts to extend this cooperative spirit throughout the hospital began almost on the first day and culminated, in the third year, in establishing the unit-team system at the hospital. In this chapter we outline the many activities of the consultants that encouraged team functioning, thus serving as forerunners of the unit-team system.

Collaboration in Individual Supervision

Individual supervision of the doctors by psychiatric consultants, the psychologists by the psychology consultant, and the psychiatric social workers by the social work consultant began in the first weeks of the project. Soon afterward, the consultants began to encourage collaboration between the doctor and psychiatric social worker responsible for a particular patient and his family. One early example of such collaborative work was that of a paranoid man whose social history revealed that his mother had kept him hidden in her house for years — an instance of *folie à deux*. The psychiatric consultant encouraged the ward physician and social worker to collaborate in the treatment and therapeutic planning for both, which they did with considerable satisfaction and success.

Collaboration in Ward Consultation

Another early collaborative attempt took the form of small-group visits to the wards, during which the consultants conferred with doctors, nurses, and psychiatric aides on difficult ward-management problems. The hospital personnel at first found the atmosphere of these ward meetings strange and disturbing, for it required a type and degrees of collaboration unique in their experience. Many of the physicians, for example, were surprised to discover that they might gain important information about a patient from talking with the nurse or psychiatric aide in attendance on the ward. Often, they were startled when a consultant sent for the patient's chart and read the nurse's notes or called in the ward attendants to discuss a patient's behavior. Such therapeutic planning conferences went even beyond the confines of the ward and included, depending upon a patient's particular needs, talks with work supervisors — in the laundry, greenhouses, or wherever.

It was only from repeated demonstrations of therapeutic gains that the staff was won over to the idea that a patient's rehabilitation depended upon his total life situation and a multitude of personal contacts within the hospital.

Collaboration in Multiple Supervision

One of the consultants who joined the team during its second year suggested an experiment in which several physicians would be supervised as a group rather than individually. Although this form of supervision never proved particularly effective in teaching basic psychodynamics and psychotherapy, it did give the doctors experience in working together, which may have helped to pave the way for their later unit-team collaboration. One of the consultant's reports alludes to such an experience in multiple supervision:

> . . . Dr. Ward, the new woman doctor, was present at the supervisory session with Drs. Willens and Craine, who both seemed eager to demonstrate to her what they knew about psychiatry. After some apparently interested listening, she began to raise some questions. . . . We went to see an elderly woman patient and discussed the possibility that the patient might be able to leave the hospital if we could obtain psychiatric social work collaboration in planning a living arrangement for her . . . Since Ward is now in charge of patients formerly taken care of by Craine, there was a good basis for discussion of these patients by the three doctors as a group. . . .

Collaboration in the Teaching Case Conferences

The teaching case conferences for the doctors regularly included the psychologist and psychiatric social worker working on the case under discussion. These conferences sometimes actually served to introduce one professional discipline to another. Dr. Burke told one of the consultants: "I never before listened to the social workers' reports; but, since the training project began, I have noticed that the consultants pay close attention to the social case history and then use it in formulating the case and planning treatment. Now I find myself listening to the social workers' reports and am surprised at how much I can learn about the patient that way."

Collaboration in Therapeutic Planning

The consultants used the case conferences to encourage interdisciplinary planning for patients, based upon the careful reconstruction of a patient's personality and pathology. Attempts were made to develop therapeutic plans that were not only flexible and appropriate for the particular patient, but could be carried out by as many of the hospital personnel as possible. Utilizing these principles (actually, ideals) of therapeutic planning tended to encourage considerable interdisciplinary teamwork. An excerpt from one of the reports demonstrates how the plan for one elderly patient could call for the teamwork of several disciplines:

> *Therapeutic Plan:* On the basis of the dynamic reconstruction of Mrs. Smith's personality and pathology, we agreed that the most advantageous form of psychotherapy, ward milieu,

and work assignment for her would include the following features:

Individual psychotherapy would probably be helpful, especially along one particular line: viz. to help her regain the ability to weep. I had the impression from my interview with her today that it might be possible to make crying much more acceptable to her, the patient herself having stated that she believes she would feel better is she could "have a good cry."

Because of her lifelong pattern of turning to men for the affection and supervision that she could never get or let herself have from women, she would probably react better to a man supervisor—one who would be rather strict with her and who would oversee her work in considerable detail (her father was strict but affectionate).

Work supervision of this kind should produce a reduction in the hallucinations of being observed in everything she does, and in the voices commenting on the mistakes she makes. Attentive and detailed supervision by a father-figure in a compatible work assignment should make these restitutive hallucinations unnecessary.

The defense of withdrawing from people could be woven into the above plan by making the work assignment one in which she was away from others for the most part: perhaps in a job at the greenhouse (she likes working with plants, and her supervisor there would be a strict man), where she could be pretty much by herself.

Some of her compulsive defense mechanisms, such as pacing back and forth, might possibly be built up in her, since they are relatively harmless forms of behavior. She herself has a great deal of conflict about the pacing, however, evidently having invested it secondarily with some of her delusional fantasies of being disturbing to and unwanted by other people. The nurses and psychiatric aides on the ward could help to make the compulsive behavior more acceptable to her, as Mrs. Fuller did recently when the patient became agitated and asked what she could do: Mrs. Fuller responded with keen intuition: "Why take a walk, Mildred!" We shall re-evaluate her response to this therapeutic plan and program in a month.

The results of the foregoing therapeutic plan were recorded in a follow-up report four months later:

Mrs. Smith's response to the treatment plan we designed for her was reviewed in the geriatric team conference today. She has shown sustained improvement as a result of this plan, even though we were unsuccessful in attempts to find a work supervisor who would be a sufficiently strict but affectionate father-figure to her. Fortunately, Mrs. Fuller has been able to provide an effective substitute for, or equivalent of, the kind of fathering that we had in mind for Mrs. Smith, so we agreed in our conference today that she should continue the same strict but affectionate approach with Mrs. Smith as before. The process of building up her previous defense of helping others is proceeding quite satisfactorily — a behavior pattern we should try to maintain in Mrs. Smith at an optimal level. We must be careful, however, not to give her *all* of the opportunities on the ward to be helpful to other patients, since other patients on the ward also need such opportunities. The geriatric team has done a splendid job in the rehabilitation of this patient, and we shall continue the therapeutic plan for Mrs. Smith very much as before.

Collaboration in Special Clinical and Research Projects

The special projects[1] were unquestionably among the most significant forerunners of team functioning at the hospital, and each of them advanced quickly in the direction of interdisciplinary collaboration. The first of these projects was the Ward Milieu Project, which was organized by a ward physician and two of his psychiatric aides and supervised by the psychology consultant. Later, Mrs. Ott, the Chief Nurse, and the nurse in charge of

[1]Reference to these projects is also made in Chapter 6, with special emphasis on their contributions to higher professional standards at the hospital.

psychiatric-aide training collaborated in extending the project to other wards. The original project therefore included four disciplines: the ward physician, psychiatric aides, nurses, and psychologist. Early in the development of this venture, the consultant wrote:

> I spent about an hour with Dr. Bernards and the two psychiatric aides . . . the project is going nicely. The group meetings are gaining more prestige with the patients, and more of them are making a point of attending. Also, the patients are beginning to use the meetings to develop plans which grow out of their discussions. Some of these plans encounter odd and, at times, very frustrating conflicts with the hospital administration. For example, I thought it might be a good idea to have small patient committees prepare snacks for the ward at night, but there is a firm rule about food on the ward . . . there was an incident at Christmas time when the patients made paper decorations, but had to take them down because they were considered a fire hazard. Now the project team is trying to arrange a fishing trip for the patients, but is afraid someone might attempt suicide by drowning! They have been warned that *any* mental patient is a suicide risk, and are leery of taking any chances. When I told them that they seem to know their patients quite well and therefore could make a good judgment about that, they were surprised that their impressions and opinions about such a matter were considered important!

In the following months, the consultant reported some morale problems on the ward milieu project that may have been due to the natural tapering-off of early gains with these very regressed patients. The ward physician evidently felt this rather strongly, for he began to withdraw somewhat from the project, behavior which drew strong criticism from the other participants. In addition, there was a tendency on the part of some members of this special project to overprotect the patients, to act maternally, rather than to enlist their active cooperation in developing plans and working them out.

By the final year of the project, however, the ward meetings were on a more substantial basis, although much exploration and groping toward solutions was necessary. It became apparent that the various unit teams were enjoying their opportunity to exchange views and experiences, were becoming less defensive about their own efforts and problems, and were working together as they had never done before. It was interesting to observe that this new attitude extended to the patients themselves:

> The "Top Chiefs" told me with considerable pride about the progress being made in instituting ward meetings throughout the hospital...
> Dr. Bolley told me later in the day that he could not see how they ever got along without ward meetings. He gave as an example the effect of such meetings upon the atmosphere of certain admission wards for disturbed patients: because of the meetings, the patients on the wards are much more concerned about and supportive toward each other. When a new patient enters the group in an agitated and disturbed state, the patients on the ward tend to take some responsi-

bility for getting him calmed down—in contrast to their former tendency to withdraw from and avoid the agitated newcomer in their midst. Dr. Bolley said that his entire unit team is impressed with how quickly the most disturbed patient will calm down when he is admitted to such a ward—within two or three hours, he claimed. ... It is interesting to note how the increased collaboration among the hospital staff appears to be reflected now in a great deal more collaborative teamwork among the patients themselves. . . .

The Geriatric Project included a physician, psychologist, social worker, nurses, activity therapists, recreation therapists, and volunteers. Before this project began, meetings were held to develop a sound plan for reading the literature on geriatric psychiatry. Equal care was given to selecting the kinds of patients and activities to be included. The team decided that the project would begin with fairly tractable patients, and later, after the accumulation of experience, would include more difficult and disturbed older people. The group was determined to avoid a "paper program," and in its approach to this difficult and interesting area of work, adopted a policy of gradual self-education that met with considerable success. One year after the project began, the consultant to the project could report:

> . . . Elizabeth Jacob, Dorothy Stock, and I went out to the hospital together to demonstrate the consultant team project to the Board of Mental Health Commissioners. . . . The various presentations went rather well, I thought. I felt par-

ticularly proud of the Geriatric Project and team. Dr. Bolley really stole the show with his down-to-earth, unselfconscious, enthusiastic description of the project, its progress, the difficulties we have faced, and our plans for the future. The Commissioners quickly caught some of the enthusiasm of this group, and took part in a lively, spirited question-and-answer discussion with the geriatric team. . . . The Commissioners were particularly impressed with the interdisciplinary composition of the geriatric team; one of them expressed admiration for the thorough multidisciplinary work-up on each patient, adding that these seemed like [Hospital X]-type work-ups.[2] Dr. Bolley replied with quiet but firm pride: "We call them *Midwest*-type work-ups, Sir." Everyone, including the Commissioners, chuckled with pleasure at the spirit and pride of this remark. . . .

The Psychopharmacology Project had dual-coordinators from the medical staff and psychology department, and also involved interdisciplinary collaboration with nurses and psychiatric aides. The doctors and nurses contributed clinical skills to the project; the psychologists provided most of the research knowledge. The project was so well organized, designed, and carried out that it was awarded a research grant from the Illinois Research and Training Authority. An excerpt from a psychiatric consultant's trip report illustrates still another dimension of the teamwork fostered by the special clinical and research

[2]Hospital X is a special hospital in the Illinois state hospital system, known for its high professional standards.

projects — collaboration among the various special-project teams:

> . . . The Psychopharmacology Project is going apace. A pharmaceutical company has heard about our project, has contacted us and offered to finance such things as secretarial help, data processing, etc. if we will test some of their drugs. The project team is rather intrigued with the idea, but will probably proceed with its plan to approach the state Research and Training Authority for a grant. The project also seems to have aroused curiosity in other quarters of the hospital itself: Dr. Bolley approached us for help in designing and carrying out a double-blind study that his team wants to do on the Geriatric Project. We invited him to sit in on our meeting, during which we spent some time discussing his project. The way he had designed the study, his group would end up not being sure whether the drug had had an actual pharmacotherapeutic or placebo effect. I debated with myself whether to just encourage him to go ahead out of his own enthusiasm, or whether to hold him in a bit and encourage him to make it a more rigorous scientific investigation. The project team took the matter into their own hands and roundly criticized his research design. He took this well, however, and accepted the psychologist's offer to help him work out a tighter experimental design.

The Alcoholic Project called for interdisciplinary collaboration among the three principal professional departments: medical, psychology, and psychiatric social work.[3] Whereas the coordinators of the Milieu and Geriatric Projects were physicians, and the Psychopharmacology Project had co-coordinators from the medical and psychology staffs, the Alcoholic Project was conceived and coordinated by the psychologist, Dr. Hoy. The fact that the leadership of these various special projects was divided among the several professional disciplines, rather than following some rigid status hierarchy, speaks well for the growth of mutual respect and team functioning among the different departmental staffs.

It may be significant that direct collaboration between the psychology and psychiatric social work staffs was the slowest to develop; these two departments had been the most competitive with each other originally; and, as noted in the following report, "Dr. Gordon, the Superintendent, felt our suggestion about collaboration between the social workers and psychologists to be an inroad on his administrative responsibilities." Here is an excerpt from the psychology consultant's final review and analysis of the consultant team project:

> The time came when we attempted to get social workers to do group therapy, along with the psychologists. This effort succeeded eventually, but ran into a major snag when it became apparent that neither the social workers themselves nor anyone else saw group therapy as a legitimate aspect of their role. When the idea was first explored with the social workers, some

[3] In fact, this project went beyond the confines of the hospital and enlisted the cooperation of friends and relatives of the alcoholic patients involved.

expressed no interest, some a fear that they would not be able to handle a therapy group. Much discussion was directed toward finding a group activity that could be regarded as appropriate to the social workers' role. When the first active effort was made—in which I was to demonstrate group discussion with patients considered ready for home care, to see whether such a session could be used in preparing patients to leave the hospital—the situation was set up by the staff in such a way that it was certain to fail: they included patients who were completely unsuitable for this purpose, some even being blind and deaf! I am not sure how much of this was due to naïveté and how much to resistance.

New Patient Orientation Meetings were settled upon eventually; but before these were well begun, Dr. Gordon sent out a memorandum canceling all such activities on the part of the social workers. He considered this collaboration of the social workers and psychologists "an inroad on his administrative responsibilities." . . . This was straightened out with the Superintendent, but upset the social workers and delayed the project. The psychologists, in the meantime, had displayed a rather condescending concern that the social workers would not be able to handle such groups. It was only after the social workers began to experience success in dealing with *groups* of patients that they themselves began to think of their work as "therapy" and began to consider using group activities that did not fall strictly within the traditional jurisdiction of social work. It was still later that actual collaboration occurred, with a social worker and psychologist acting as cotherapists. . . .

It was late in the second year of the consultant team project that these two departments joined forces effectively to organize and carry out the New Patient Orientation Project. Once this collaboration was established, it became a potent force in the later unit teams, supporting the doctors (especially the Unit Chiefs) in a humanistic, psychological approach to patients' problems.

Collaboration in Special Training Projects

Considerably less interdisciplinary collaboration took place in the special training projects than in the research projects, but some crossing of professional boundaries did occur, and this may therefore have represented an additional forerunner of team functioning. The interdisciplinary aspects of these special training projects warrant a brief description.

The Volunteers Project demanded the most significant interdisciplinary collaboration: that between the doctors and the volunteers. Prior to instituting this project, essentially no collaboration existed between the medical staff and the Volunteer Services Department of the hospital. The following excerpts from a consultant's trip report highlights its collaborative aspects.

The Clinical Director and I met with the Unit Chiefs, who hadn't the faintest notion why we were going to meet with volunteers! We had quite a discussion about the role of volunteers in the hospital, which they knew little or nothing about. Dr. Christy asked me pointedly: "But what are they going to do for us?" I answered just as pointedly: "For once, you are going to do something for *them!*" Rather than resenting this, they seemed moderately pleased at the idea. I told them they would be helping the volunteers in training by answering questions for them — that this was a new group having their indoctrination training. The Director of Volunteer Services had assembled a rather large group of volunteers for our meeting. I took the first questions, giving very simple answers and explanations, and stressing always that they should be concerned with the healthy side of the patient. As the questions about the hospital became more detailed, I turned them over to each of the doctors in turn. They gave good answers and explanations, and even their English seemed to improve as they talked! The questions went on and on, and when it came time to go, the doctors actually seemed reluctant to leave. . . .

Other special training projects were organized and carried out — in each case at the request of staff groups within the hospital — for four hospital departments: a training program for nurses, for activity therapists, for psychiatric aides, and for the Protestant chaplain. The principal collaborative aspect of these special training programs was the fact that the professional disciplines of the consultants conducting these projects differed from those of the trainees, which may have had some effect in promoting collaborative teamwork among the various departmental staffs within the hospital.

Two other aspects of the special training projects may also have encouraged interdisciplinary collaboration, although in rather indirect ways. One was that consultants who undertook the leadership of special training projects did so by reducing the amount of time they devoted to training other hospital staff groups: one consultant dropped his case conference with the doctors in order to spend more time in teaching the nurses. Changes of this kind were discussed with the hospital staff—although the decisions were not always arrived at as collaboratively as they might have been—and each such change produced definite effects upon the staff. The staff group from whom training time had been taken were hurt and angry; the groups receiving additional time responded with pleasure and pride. These reactions were always temporary, however, and never very intense. Shifts of this kind drew everyone's attention to the so-called "ancillary" departments and may have prompted collaboration in the form of "sharing" the consultants.

Key staff members were encouraged to carry out as much of the special training as possible, and this policy also had collaborative significance. For example, in the training of activity therapists, a psychiatric consultant supervised a psychologist, who in turn taught the activity therapists. The special training programs have continued along the original lines, for the most part, but toward the end of the Midwest project were gradually being absorbed into the unit teams.

The coordinator of the Illinois-City consultant team, the Superintendent, and I did some talking about the future of the special projects. The special training projects for nurses, activity therapists, chaplains, psychiatric aides, and volunteers will be integrated gradually into the unit teams as ongoing, in-service training programs. The special clinical and research projects, on the other hand, will probably be continued with consultant supervision from the Illinois-City team....

Collaboration Involving the Hospital Administration

By "the hospital administration" we refer to three top administrative officers of the hospital: the Superintendent, Assistant Superintendent, and Clinical Director. In discussing team functioning as it involves these "Top Chiefs," a distinction must be made between communication and collaboration. A great deal of communication went on between the Chicago and Illinois-City consultant teams, on the one hand, and the hospital administration, on the other; but there was considerably less collaboration, i.e., meangingful, fruitful interchange of ideas and sharing of decisions. As for the relationship of the "Top Chiefs" to the hospital staff, both communication and collaboration have remained continuing problems.

Such a gulf between the administration and clinical staff of a state hospital is common enough, but the experience of one such institution has shown that the relationship between the two need not be so distant and vertically hierarchical: at the Utah State Hospital, the Superintendent, Dr. Owen P. Heninger (1963), was successful in bringing about far greater collaboration through the administrative decentralization of his hospital. In most such settings, however, the chief administrative officers are set apart from the rest of the staff, much as the General Officer Corps of the army is set apart from all other ranks, officers and enlisted men alike.

It should be noted that the later administration of Midwest State Hospital was much less isolated from the clinical staff than the previous one was. The second Superintendent, Dr. Fisher, helped to institute and actively supported the unit-team system, whereas the previous Superintendent kept the various hospital departments functionally separated from each other and individually responsible solely to himself. The second Assistant Superintendent, Dr. Owens, was active in direct clinical work with individual patients, whereas the previous Assistant Superintendent was completely divorced from clinical responsibilities. The eventual Clinical Director, Dr. Simon, was trained in psychiatry and neurology by our consultant team, and he attempted to promote interdisciplinary collaboration—horizontally, at least, among the staff—wherever possible.

Still, there was an ever-present necessity for the "Top Chiefs" of the hospital to be preoccupied with problems concerning the hospital's relationship to the community at large, and to a hierarchy of state officials in particular. Much of their energy was consumed by minor, occasionally major, crises concerning community reactions to the hospital and by maintaining administrative peace with state officials. This may account in part for the inadequate communication with the clinical staff and consultants of a state hospital.

From another standpoint, and in all fairness to the hospital administration, the consultant team failed at the outset to establish a sufficiently collaborative model for its relationship with the chief administrative officers of the hospital, and from that failure sprang many problems. We quote from the minutes of one of the consultant team's monthly planning meetings.

Discussion developed along the lines of the difficulties, disappointments, and frustrations we encountered in attempting to establish working rapprochement with the hospital administration—primarily the top administration. Until Dr. Fisher became Superintendent, we never really achieved such an alliance with them; the previous chiefs allowed us to work parallel to, but not with them. Although the team's policies and activities were all cleared *through* the Superintendent, we never succeeded in getting him interested and involved enough in the training program so that he would work *with* us and assume responsibility for the project. The question arose whether it would not be advisable in our second project to institute meetings with the top administration before the more general educational program is begun. Such meetings at the outset of the project might help to establish the principle and policy of the consultant team's working collaboratively with the administration and of the hospital administration's being actively, responsibly involved in the training program rather than simply going along with it.

Our failure to establish such a working alliance at Midwest no doubt contributed to phenomena such as the original Superintendent's hiring of another psychiatric consultant and his trying to arrange courses in psychology for the doctors at a local college, without discussing either plan with us.... To achieve effective rapport, everything should be discussed

> with and channeled through the administrative
> heads of the hospital.... The administrative
> heads have to be given a measure of responsi-
> bility for carrying out the team's work.

This principle was not followed effectively in the early stages of the Midwest venture, an error not repeated in the second state hospital project.

The most significant achievements in collaboration between the consultant team and hospital administration occurred in connection with the formation and functioning of the Journal Club and the Education Committee, the organization of the Illinois-City consultant team, and the reorganization of the hospital and staff into three smaller units and interdisciplinary unit teams. The most effective, though still spotty and difficult, collaboration occurred in connection with the unit-team system, which the new Superintendent took immediate steps to implement upon his arrival. These necessary, rapid, administrative actions resulted in several serious difficulties, however: incomplete understanding of the goals and methods of the unit-team system; insufficient planning of the change-over to a drastically different kind of organization; and inadequate preparation of the staff to meet this major hospital reorganization. A great deal of *ex post facto* collaboration between the consultant teams, the administration, and the staff was necessary to straighten out the problems produced by insufficient preplanning and trial runs of the new program.

Even before the unit system began operating, it had effects upon the hospital personnel. Confusion was evident throughout the hospital, and there was much discussion about which team had the best personnel and which the most attractive space. A few days after the new system was introduced, a psychiatric consultant reported:

The doctors wanted to talk about the unit teams.... A great deal of skepticism was expressed. Dr. Bolley felt that there was a need for a coordinated physical set-up for the infirmary, which was not available under this plan. Dr. Bernards wanted to know if there was any literature on the subject. Someone said that the staff seemed to be under much tension because they didn't know what to expect. There was the somewhat resigned feeling, however, that this might lead to better communication.

A week later, another consultant observed: "No one seems to be quite sure what the unit system means, although most seem to feel that, like the open door policy and drugs, it is a good thing." And the next month, the team coordinator reported: "So far as the unit system is concerned, I think things are going about as one would expect. I feel we can do little more than give moral support during this turbulent period and encourage Dr. Fisher to make himself available for the guidance and support of the unit-team staffs."

Several months after the new system was introduced and after a great deal of "postplanning" that ideally should have been done in advance, the unit teams were functioning well. But problems of collaboration between the Unit Chiefs and the administration persisted:

> ... Two of the Unit Chiefs said that the problems they have now are not within the unit team itself, which is functioning smoothly and efficiently, but with the "Top Chiefs." They explained that the administration sometimes makes decisions about patients which the unit team feels to be matters for its own decision.

Actually, I think this mild tension is normal, natural, and inevitable in some respects. I don't believe that the "Top Chiefs" really have any wish or need to undercut the authority of the unit teams. In all probability, they intercede at times because of certain pressures on them from the outside which require some action.... The real problem is, once again, a deficiency of communication.

The problems of collaboration between the administration and consultant team were intensified by the change-over from the Chicago to the Illinois-City team. Although difficulties of this kind existed between the administration and the I-C team, the final trip report of the Chicago team had a more optimistic tone:

Possibly the most important matter that came up at this meeting was the discussion about planning a curriculum in basic psychiatry for the four new doctors. Before my eyes, I saw the beginnings of a real collaboration between the hospital administration and the I-C team in planning a coordinated curriculum that would involve conferences and seminars, not only by the consultants, but also by the Superintendent, Assistant Superintendent, and Clinical Director. If this kind of cooperation can be affected, a new and potentially permanent foundation for the training project may have been established at the hospital.

CHAPTER FIVE

Social Systems Changes

THE MIDWEST PROJECT CAN BE THOUGHT OF in terms of an encounter between two social systems: the hospital and the consulting team. Of these, the hospital was a permanent system, already in existence for many years before the consultants arrived and certainly destined to outlive their term of service. In contrast, the consultant team was a temporary system with a predetermined three-year life span,[1] constructed for the sole purpose of interacting with the hospital in order to influence or change it.[2]

In the beginning, the team did not think of itself or the hospital as a system, but felt its mission to be one of teaching individuals. Soon, however, members of the team

[1]The three-year duration of the project was based upon fairly arbitrary considerations—possibly also some irrelevant ones, such as the fact that most residency programs in psychiatry are for three-year periods. We wanted to have enough time at the hospital to develop and carry out training programs in some detail, but at the same time wanted to complete our training activities within "a few years" so we could move on to other state hospitals needing such help. A period of three years seemed a reasonable compromise between these two objectives. In retrospect, this length of time still seems about right for a consultant team project of this kind.

[2]This way of looking at the hospital and the team was suggested by M. B. Miles, Ed., in *Innovation in Education* (N.Y.: Bureau of Public., Teachers College, Columbia Univ., 1964).

began to be aware of the hospital as a system, with established goals, practices, and customs, which, like the individuals within the structure, could influence and be · influenced by the consultants' teaching efforts.

Of necessity, this account of the interaction between the permanent system of the hospital and the temporary system of the consulting team must be undertaken from the point of view of the consultants. Moreover, the team never systematically studied the hospital's organizational structure or its own. Rather, the consultants continually made informal observations which they wrote down. It is from these rich though incomplete impressions on their regular trip reports that this view of two systems has been reconstructed, in an attempt to understand the experience in organizational terms. It seems in retrospect that otherwise puzzling events occurring during these years take on meaning if they are understood in terms of the mutual impact of two social systems.

Looking back, it seems clear that the consultants made a number of assumptions about the hospital and the nature of the task there. These had to do with the goals of the hospital and of the consulting project, and of the structure required to achieve those goals.

That the goal of the hospital was to provide care and treatment of mental patients;

That this goal was, or should be, achieved through the integrated efforts of the physicians, social workers, psychologists, nurses, and other personnel at the hospital;

That each of these disciplines was, or should be, characterized by clearly defined, differentiated, and complementary roles (the doctors having primary authority and responsibility for medical care of patients; the social workers dealing with personal histories and the patients' families; the psychologists handling diagnostic testing, etc.);

That the goal of the encounter between the hospital and the team was to improve patient care through improving the knowledge and skills of all the professional personnel;

That any changes resulting from the consulting program could not be expected to be self-sustaining, and that therefore a replacement team would be necessary at the end of the project.

The first assumption was taken for granted by all concerned, consulting team and hospital alike. Yet it proved to be a vastly oversimplified statement of the hospital's goals, for it assumed that a single, overriding, and shared goal existed at the hospital and dominated its activities.

The second and third assumptions were implicit and seemed verified by the official organizational structure of the hospital: the physicians functioned as ward managers and chaired intake and evaluation staff meetings; the psychologists and social workers assumed the tasks traditionally expected of them; the hospital was divided into departments of psychology, social service, nursing, etc., each with its own chief. Although the hospital and team accepted this traditional form as characteristic of most psychiatric units throughout the country, the fact was that, as in most state hospitals, a quite different and more complex organizational structure actually existed.

The fourth assumption was explicitly accepted by the

consulting team and the hospital (meaning, in this case, the Superintendent, Clinical Director, and Department Heads). Everyone agreed that the goal of the project was to improve patient care by helping the professional personnel, especially the doctors, to improve their skills. Other goals and other forms of encounter between the consultants and the hospital were not anticipated at this time.

The final assumption was explicit, at least within the team, where it was understood from the beginning that an effort would be made to recruit a local team to replace the Chicago group at the end of three years.

It is not surprising that among the first things the consultants began to notice were features of the hospital manifestly inconsistent with the fact or spirit of these assumptions, as can be seen by an examination of the trip reports of the first three or four months:

The doctors were abysmally insecure in every respect, except that of dealing with physical illness. Their uncertainty extended to prescribing medication for psychiatric problems as well as to ward management. Some of them feared and avoided direct contact with patients. In general, the doctors, especially the new ones, derived little satisfaction from their professional roles in the hospital; many of them planned to leave as soon as they could. Further, they were isolated from the outside community, medical and otherwise.

The various hospital departments tended to avoid and withdraw from one another. Psychology and social work operated according to strict jurisdictional rules sanctioned by the administration. It was regarded as inappropriate for psychologists to see members of a family or for social workers to conduct therapy. The social workers seemed to derive greatest satisfaction from their

Family Care Program, and were oriented primarily toward raising the hospital's discharge rate.

The psychologists were frustrated in their roles as diagnosticians because they felt the doctors ignored their diagnostic reports; they were frustrated in their role as therapists because their accomplishments did not match their goal of "deep," reconstructive therapy. Both the psychologists and the social workers were producing less than their best work.

Some of the aides seemed only to wish to be left alone with their chronic, withdrawn patients. Others, who were more active, behaved too maternally toward their patients or were primarily interested in maintaining a "good," i.e., orderly ward. Some of the aides were frustrated because they wanted more contact with and direction from the doctors.

Morale was poor and self-esteem seemed low among many of the personnel, some of whom displayed a punitive, contemptuous attitude toward patients. The working day was marked by long lunch hours and coffee breaks. Social workers and psychologists were frequently absent in order to give talks to church and civic groups. The personnel regarded the Superintendent and Clinical Director as people to be "gotten around," cajoled, or manipulated. There was almost no straightforward discussion of matters of mutual concern. The Superintendent and Clinical Director expressed contempt toward the doctors and other personnel for what they called "their laziness." The hospital administration was preoccupied with gaining favorable publicity for the hospital, making a good impression on the community, and, above all, guarding against any episode that might lead to criticism of the hospital.

Some effective work was accomplished, but it tended

to occur in isolated pockets of the hospital—an occasional ward program, the social workers' efforts in the Family Care Program, some of the therapeutic work conducted by the psychologists, one or two kindly doctors who maintained good contact with their patients, the Activity Therapy Program, and others. The over-all performance of the hospital in its task of evaluating and treating patients was poor. Patients tended to get "lost" within the hospital; many patients received no more than custodial care; more intensive treatment, when it occurred, was undertaken haphazardly; and staff members working with the same patient often did not communicate and consequently worked at cross purposes.

At first, the consultants found it difficult to make sense of these observations. Because the hospital did not display the *expected* organization, it was easy to assume that there was *no* organization. The early impression was one of chaos relieved by seemingly random examples of good functioning. The hospital seemed to be functioning badly with reference to what the consultants assumed to be not only its most important, but its sole goal—that of providing good patient care.

Understandably, the team spent much more time and energy observing the hospital than observing itself. But as time went on, some self-scrutiny became essential as differences in approach made themselves evident. For example, there were different ideas about how much time should be devoted to the hospital during a consulting day; there were varying views on whether personnel other than doctors should be permitted to attend the morning seminars; later, there were disagreements about the value of group supervision for the doctors. Observations about the hospital did not always match, and some team members became concerned about issues that seemed of little importance to others. These intrateam problems, however, never became critical because the team members respected one another and enjoyed working together.

Planning for the consulting program was largely in the hands of the consultants, and theirs was an empirical approach: what worked was continued; what didn't work was abandoned, changed, or (if it was regarded as essential) maintained in the face of objections. Throughout the project years, the interaction of the team and the hospital had a "play-it-by-ear" flavor. The curriculum, representing as it did a consensus among the team members about what would be useful activity, had an underlying coherence and consistency. But, at the same time, larger and smaller modifications were continually made in response to events at the hospital and to the reactions of the people being taught.

Both the hospital and the consultant team changed as a result of their encounter with one another. For the hospital, the system changes involved two new organizational features which had far-reaching effects on its character: the unit teams and the emergence of the special projects.[3] For the team, perhaps the most important change was in its increased appreciation of the complexity of the mental hospital as an organization, and in its revised ideas about teaching in such a setting. Some of these changes merit further elaboration.

The Hospital as a System

If the consulting team was at first inclined to see the situation at the hospital as one of chaos with a few bright spots of effective functioning, this view was derived from an

---

[3]These results of the interaction of hospital and consulting team are discussed in detail in Chapter 6.

imperfect understanding of the hospital. The hospital was indeed characterized by a structure that made sense, though it was not the one the team expected or valued.

When we started, both groups could agree that the goal of the hospital was to provide effective patient care, and that this meant accurate and prompt diagnosis, appropriate treatment, and discharge whenever possible. But whereas the hospital seemed to place major emphasis on curing and discharging patients, the consultants added a stress on improving the life of the patient while he remained within the hospital. Both groups recognized that a large number of patients would never be able to leave; the team felt interested in these patients, the hospital felt frustrated by them.

The goals "assumed" at the start of the project would, three years later, have to be almost entirely restated, this time according to *whose* goals they might be. For the staff doctors, the primary goal was a personal one, not very much related to the hospital itself. Their need was to survive in drastically altered circumstances and to maintain as best they could their personal sense of worth. For the hospital administration, the maintenance of prestige and a good reputation in the community seemed of great importance. The administration was also very interested in increasing the hospital's discharge rate. In this they were joined by Social Service, which was strongly committed to its program of family care. Much of the social workers' sense of self-esteem and accomplishment seemed to stem from their success in placing patients on family care or arranging for their discharge. The psychology staff, in contrast, appeared to value above all else the conduct of psychotherapy that had an intensive, uncovering character. The aides, and to some extent the nurses, seemed to value neatly kept wards and well-behaved patients. In this, some goals coincided with or reinforced one another, while others were in conflict. For example, in working toward the discharge of a patient, the social workers (under pressure from the administration, transmitted through the staff physicians) might interfere with a psychologist's efforts at prolonged in-patient therapy. The doctors' personal preoccupations at times diverted their energies from activities related to patient care. When certain of the goals remained implicit and unclarified, the personnel became baffled and behaved as if they were lazy, resistant, or uninterested. Further, some of the individual goals, and even some of the shared goals, could not realistically be met. The psychologists may have wished to conduct psychotherapy of an intensive, uncovering character, but with a population of chronic, regressed patients, suitable candidates for such psychotherapy were hard to find, and when they were found they would very likely be regarded as suitable for discharge by other personnel and would soon leave the hospital. It was difficult for the hospital administration to satisfy its need for prestige and recognition when so important a group as the physicians was not equipped for its job. Even the shared goal of increasing the discharge rate could be achieved only in a limited way because of the presence of so many chronic and aged patients, many of whom had been in the hospital for ten to forty years.

The team's original assumption that the hospital was a single system organized to achieve the goal of providing patient care was a gross oversimplification. In fact, a multiplicity of goals was present, some having nothing to do with patient care. Many of these goals could not, by the nature of the situation, be met, and some were mutually incompatible. Although the hospital personnel seemed to accept the prevailing view of the proper organization and conduct of a psychiatric unit, with each discipline performing its essential but limited activities in relation to patients, this traditional form of organization could not really function, primarily because of the inexperience and lack of training of the doctors. Though nominally in charge, the doctors were less qualified for the work expected of them than were the psychologists, social workers, and other staff. Typically, the psychologist or social worker was better prepared to understand a particular patient, yet did not have ultimate responsibility for him. On his side, the doctor could derive little self-esteem from his work, and it is understandable that he tended to concentrate on the physical ills of patients, withdrawing from other forms of direct contact with them and from other personnel as well. The doctors were in the most difficult position, psychologically, of any of the personnel, because they felt most strongly the frustrations, anxieties, and lowered self-esteem associated with knowing they were unequipped for their task.

The situation was also difficult for the psychologists and social workers. They were frustrated in their wish to work with the doctors, to contribute to their mutual task, and to have their work understood and appreciated. Often, though they were aware of being able to make sounder decisions than the doctors, they were stopped by the knowledge that to do so would mean increasing their self-esteem at the expense of the doctors and facing the reality that the ideal system was not the current one. Both groups responded similarly by allowing work standards to deteriorate and by seeking satisfying and esteem-building activities outside the hospital. Lecturing to various civic and church groups undoubtedly offered the psychologists and social workers welcome opportunities to escape the frustrating hospital environment and to increase self-esteem through displaying professional expertise. This flight by the social workers and psychologists was supported by the hospital administration, for whom it was a means of increasing the hospital's prestige in the community.

In an effort to account for the failure to meet goals without feeling responsible, the staff indulged in a great deal of accusation and recrimination: the hospital administration blamed the doctors and others for being lazy; the psychologists expressed anger at the social workers for their lack of cooperation; the psychologists and social workers were angry at the Clinical Director for not conducting meetings properly; and everyone came down hard on the less adequate members of the staff.

Because preferred procedures for working together as a team could not be put into effect, the hospital developed substitute procedures for accomplishing basic work with patients. Lip service was paid to the official hierarchy, but in actual practice the official lines of authority and responsibility were bypassed. The Clinical Director sat in on all meetings, and it was he, rather than the ward physicians, who made the final decisions about diagnosis and discharge. In selecting patients for group therapy, the psychologists consulted not the doctors, but the ward attendants. Because the aides could not get help from the doctors, they tended to seek out the Head Nurse for advice about patients. Thus the necessary work of the hospital was accomplished at some loss of efficiency and reduction of standards. But by looking—as the team did at first—in the places where one expected to see this work accomplished, one saw nothing, for the work occurred at the interstices of the official organization.

A mode of communication existed within the hospital that was characterized by mutual avoidance among the various disciplines, but continuous and close communication within each discipline. In addition, certain substitutive channels of communication were used heavily—for example, between psychologists and certain aides, between aides and nurses, between the Superintendent and Clinical Director. Communication between the various disciplines was thus rendered less necessary, but the mutual avoidance may also have functioned to control interdepartmental hostility and resentment: the doctors, psychologists, and social workers blamed one another from a distance. Lack of communication also made it easier to maintain the fiction that the official lines of authority, competence, and responsibility were real. If the aides never consulted the doctors about their difficult patients, they avoided confrontation with the fact that the doctors could be of little help.

It is possible that the contemptuous, punitive attitudes toward the patients on the part of some hospital personnel might have been a device for separating staff from patients. Perhaps the patients served as a convenient target for the expression of frustration and anger.

The Consultant Team as a System

When the project began, the consultant team was a new group whose members had to find ways of planning together, dealing with disagreements among themselves, and maintaining morale and commitment. Looking back, it seems evident that the team developed a characteristic way of operating. First of all, it tolerated individual differences. If two people disagreed strongly about a procedure, both ways might be tried. It was taken for granted that each consultant might want to proceed with his preceptees or conduct the teaching conferences in his own way.

It talked issues out during breakfast meetings, both formal matters related to the teaching program, and short-term, often personal problems and complaints. Though these matters added to already overburdened agendas, discussion of them almost certainly paid off in maintaining morale and communication.

The team exercised a certain amount of suppression of conflict. Sometimes disagreements were resolved by withdrawal from the field by a team member who felt less strongly about the issue or who felt himself to have less influence. By adopting this solution, the team may sometimes have paid the price of a temporary reduction of involvement on the part of one of its members.

Members of the team developed mutual respect for one another as persons and as professionals. In this important area, the team was most fortunate: no one was regarded as a problem child, and the expectation was that no one would make any serious mistakes. A continuing mutual respect and confidence made room for consider-able individual differences and the free expression of preferences and opinions.

A differentiation of roles and personalities gradually evolved within the team. For example, the team members grew to expect that one member would always push his ideas insistently, but always in the last instance listen to the others, and that another member would try to resolve conflict both within the team and between team and hospital staff. Such knowledge of one another was useful in the face-to-face contacts at breakfast meetings and in interpreting colleagues' written reports.

Much of what went on during the early months of the project could be understood in terms of two systems'—hospital and team—attempting to use each other to create or maintain a preferred situation. Planning was largely in the hands of the consultants. This meant that the project was structured around the team's image of the well-functioning hospital, stressing the psychiatric skills of the doctors, pressuring the psychologists to produce diagnostic reports based on testing rather than interviewing, and generally aiming toward a different division of labor from that existing. By continually pointing out the value of communication, the team was attempting to encourage interdisciplinary decision-making. By working hard and continually throughout the day, the team was attempting to press the hospital toward greater commitment to professional work.

At the same time, members of the staff were exerting pressure to get the consultants' help in maintaining the existing character and practices of the hospital. Staff members frequently asked one or another of the consultants to intervene for them with the Superintendent, or to cooperate in some indirect plan for influencing the hospital administration. The administration subtly pressed the consultants to perceive the doctors as they did—as a "lazy, incompetent lot." The administration also pressed the consultants to activities that might improve the hospital's prestige in the community—radio programs, forums, and the like. For the most part, the hospital personnel tried to maintain its previous character and structure through passive resistance: It took a long time for the consultants to get the personnel to talk to one another about patients, and an early attempt to press the doctors and aides to engage in ward-milieu projects fell apart.

Because the two systems clung to such different models of hospital organization, much of their early interaction was characterized by mutual pressuring, active or passive attempts to resist the influence, and giving in or giving up. That the project succeeded in spite of this state of affairs is probably owing to several factors. First, the hospital personnel, while exerting strenuous efforts to maintain the status quo, nevertheless clearly indicated dissatisfaction with it. It was as if the staff had evolved its practices, not from preference, but from necessity, as compromise solutions. There was a feeling of resignation about the situation, and an important early response to the team was increase in hope and optimism. Merely by selecting this hospital for its project, the team communicated a feeling that change and improvement were possible. The curriculum itself communicated the expectation that the doctors could learn psychiatry, the hospital personnel could learn to work together more effectively, and patient care could be improved. Thus, the hospital seemed ready to change should changed conditions make this possible, and they were encouraged in this direction by the consultants.

A second important factor was the interaction of staff members. Whereas the consultants were naïve in their understanding of the hospital's organizational structure, they were very understanding of individuals encountered there and ready to understand the pressures and anxieties under which the staff members labored. Once the consultants became well acquainted with the staff, it was possible to express this understanding and use it in teaching and supervision. As the consultants began to help the various people on the staff deal with their anxieties, feelings of trust and liking developed between members of the team and those with whom they worked directly. The development of such a relationship was far more difficult with members of the hospital administration. In the case of the original Superintendent, where a close personal relationship never developed, the team failed for a long time to empathize with his difficulties and tended to interpret his behavior as stubbornness. On the whole, however, the team's ability and eagerness to work individually with the staff could be traced to past training. All the team members were accustomed to dealing with individuals rather than with a large social entity like a hospital. It is understandable that the route to resolving tensions proceeded from one encounter to another. A good example lay in the team's pressure upon the doctors to conduct psychotherapy, in the face of much fear and resistance. Once a doctor began working with a single patient, his preceptor was gentle and understanding in helping him to deal both with the patient and with his own anxieties. But by pressing these doctors to a radical shift in their roles vis-à-vis the patients, the consultants were in fact interfering with an institutional pattern of withdrawal from patients. This pattern of withdrawal had been adopted by a large segment of the hospital's personnel, which had shifted roles in accommodation to it. By helping the doctors to assume this hitherto avoided activity, the consultants were not only helping them to learn psychotherapy, but paving the way for widespread institutional changes.

In its immediate response to expressions of personal interest among the staff, the team was able to translate into action many long-dormant ideas. This often took the form of dissolving blockages to action, either from within hospital personnel themselves or in the hospital environment. When the Geriatric Project was just beginning, the Superintendent complained about the slowness of its progress, attributing this to the laziness of the doctor in charge. The team's consultant to the project firmly endorsed its pace, insisting that a thorough survey of the hospital's geriatric population and a review of the literature would pay off later. By taking this position, he protected the doctor from the full impact of the Superintendent's criticism and reduced the chances that the project might be scuttled. Such an action influenced the hospital system in several ways. It introduced a perception that ran counter to the administration's prevailing view of the doctors; rather than agreeing that the doctor was lazy, the consultant saw him as displaying prudent and appropriate behavior. It also made possible a new and lasting entity—the Geriatric Project—and set up a model of interdisciplinary functioning that could be observed by others.

The entire history of the interaction of hospital and consulting team could probably be summed up in terms of the long series of transactions between a consultant and individuals or groups from the hospital staff. Each of these transactions had some wide impact on the character or structure of the hospital. The widening circle of impact was in itself a demonstration that a coherent and interdependent social system existed at the hospital, for if the situation had been merely chaotic, dealing with a single person would have affected only that person.

This view of the project as the interplay of two systems raises related questions. (1) In what way did the assumptions the consultants made at the beginning of the project influence the course of the project? (2) Would it have been useful had the consultants better understood the nature of the two systems and their interaction while the project was underway?

To the first question one might say that, by making certain assumptions about goals and procedures at the hospital, the consulting team was led to omit exploring and checking out these assumptions. Some early actions thus had to be revised later, piecemeal, and in response to problems. Also, because the team accepted at face value verbal agreements about the major goal of the consulting program, other important goals were overlooked. The team assumed, for example, that changes could be maintained only with the aid of a replacement consulting team, an assumption that doubtless influenced the entire project and ignored the possibility that the hospital itself could introduce systems changes for its own continued education.[4]

In answer to the second question, had the consultant team been aware of some characteristics of the hospital system, the project might have begun with less confusion and greater acceptance by the hospital personnel. The team was inclined to disapprove of things which were in fact functional for the hospital. Had this been better understood, the consultants might have handled their negative reactions more easily and would certainly have modified some of the original "package deal" approach to

---

[4]In the second state hospital project, rather than replacing itself with a local consultant team, the Chicago team encouraged and helped the hospital staff to develop its own Education Committee, with responsibilities for planning, coordinating, and carrying out teaching and training activities throughout the hospital.

planning. As it was, collaborative planning was minimal, without an opportunity to share feelings, goals, or assumptions. If the team had been unable to modify its activities throughout the three years, had it insisted on carrying out its original plan, the project would almost certainly have fallen into stereotyped routine and been far less successful.[5]

The goal of a consultant project is not, of course, to learn about the systems characteristics of the hospital, the team, or the encounter between them. But failure to attend to these characteristics may lead both sides to operate on a "fallen from grace" approach vis-à-vis the other. Whatever does not fit one's own assumptions or needs is seen as a defect, disapproved of, and scheduled for change or eradication. Much otherwise avoidable stress ensues with such an approach. While an understanding of systems characteristics does not in itself teach psychiatry, it may help to create conditions under which psychiatry is more readily learned.

[5]The experience at Midwest led the second state hospital team to begin its project in quite a new way, with much more collaborative preplanning between the two systems, and provision for an ongoing steering committee composed of members of both systems.

CHAPTER SIX

Results: A General Summary

IT IS DIFFICULT TO KNOW or to even guess at all of the results of the project or of their permanence. That the three years had a considerable impact is unquestionable, however, and this chapter deals with some of the most evident results from the viewpoints of both the hospital and the consultant team.

Effects upon Morale

Soon after the consultant team arrived, a change in the morale of the hospital staff could be observed. This was particularly true of the doctors, psychologists, and psychiatric social workers, who became more optimistic and enthusiastic about their work, less discouraged and apathetic. Since almost any innovation at a state hospital may produce such an effect temporarily, this mood shift was noteworthy only in its permanence; it continued throughout the three years of the project, survived the change-over to a local team of consultants, continued during the four-year tenure of the local consultant team, and was still evident some years after that.

This result surprised the consultants, who had anticipated some disappointment and disillusionment when it
became clear that they brought no "magic" from Chicago.
Morale continued to build up, however, eventually becoming consolidated as a new and more confident outlook
on the possibilities, as well as the problems, of state
hospital work. One of the most significant measures of the
new confidence was in the number of staff physicians who
decided to stay at the hospital and make a career of state
hospital psychiatry. Approximately three-fourths of the
doctors who were involved in the training programs of the
Chicago and Illinois-City consultant teams remained at
Midwest and planned to continue their training as psychiatrists. This trend stands in sharp contrast to the previous
rapid turnover of doctors at the hospital.

Some observations and comments by one of the I-C
consultants about a new doctor at the hospital may
illustrate this change in outlook:

> ...I had a most interesting individual confer-
> ence with Dr. Ricky, the new doctor. Ricky is fif-
> ty-eight years old and came to this country from
> Central Europe in 1948. He described his diffi-
> culties in learning the language, studying to get
> his medical license, working at another Illinois
> state hospital, then at Midwest Hospital. He left
> this hospital to go into private (general) practice
> just before the Chicago consultant team began
> working here. The attempt at private practice
> was short-lived. He found that to support himself,
> he had to work very long hours, taking jobs as a
> part-time physician in industrial plants during
> the daytime and seeing private patients in the
> evenings. He returned to Midwest recently with

the idea of "retiring," as he called it, and "taking life easy." He was quite shaken by the changes he observed when he returned. Whereas he had hoped to be given an easy assignment such as he had before, treating the diabetics, epileptics, and flat feet at the hospital, he found himself exposed to one of the new unit teams and surrounded by a strange kind of excitement about psychiatry on the part of the other doctors, from which he felt left out. He feels discouraged and unable to learn a new specialty at his age, saying forlornly: "I just don't understand this dynamic psychiatry...."

[Four months later] ... The next conference was with Dr. Ricky. I am surprised and delighted at his growing interest in psychiatry. Evidently he has not been able to resist the contagious excitement of the other doctors about psychiatry. He brought a copy of Noyes and Kolb's *Modern Clinical Psychiatry* to the conference with him; he has begun plowing through it from beginning to end and has already finished about a hundred pages. This man, who thought he would come back and hide in the state hospital where he worked before, is developing a real interest in psychiatry and is learning something about this field for the first time, even though he worked here previously for seven years! He brought the Noyes and Kolb book to the conference because he cannot understand some of the words and technical terms. We agreed that I will tutor him. He will mark the doubtful words and passages as he reads them, and in his conferences with me I

shall try to interpret and explain them to
him. . . .

[Eight months after Dr. Ricky's return to the
hospital] . . . I had a most interesting discussion
with Dr. Ricky about his reading of Noyes and
Kolb. He has now read the book three times. The
first reading was quite difficult, for most of his
time was spent looking up unfamiliar words in
the dictionary and then returning to the text to
fit the meaning and pronunciation into the context of what he was reading. The second and
third readings made increasingly more sense to
him. His clinical work is making slow but steady
progress, too. . . . It is fascinating to observe the
growth of this fifty-eight-year-old physician's interest in and knowledge about psychiatry. He
said today that he feels he has started a new
career. . . .

What was it about the project that produced such
striking and apparently permanent changes in the morale
of the hospital staff? Although the question cannot be
answered with certainty, two possible contributing factors
might be mentioned. One was the fairly consistent enthusiasm and optimistic outlook of the consultant team, as evidenced by the following progress and trip reports, the first
dating from three months after the project began:

. . . It is too early to tell what the effects of this
program may be in helping to raise the professional standards and improve patient care at the
hospital. At the present time, we can report
more about the effects of the project upon the
consultants than upon the hospital personnel

and patients. All of the consultants are enthusiastic about the project, find it highly interesting, and are optimistic about its future. . . .

[And after one year] We hope the focus of this report upon the activities of the consultant team will not give an erroneous impression that we consider ourselves responsible for most of the progress at Midwest State Hospital during the past year. Although the consultant team organized itself originally with the goal of trying to "help out" in a remote state hospital, we are not at all certain whether they or we have benefited most from the project. The experience has been a rich and rewarding one both professionally and personally for all of us on the consultant team. The staff, personnel, and patients at the hospital have taught us many things we could not have learned in any other way. . . .

[After two years] . . . In reviewing our work at Midwest State Hospital during the second year of the project, we have the impression that the project is a healthy one and is achieving its main goals. As we have gained experience, the strain of the work during our first year has decreased considerably. Travel to and from the hospital during bad weather continues to be a serious problem, but one which the determination and enthusiasm of the consultant team have been able to surmount. In our two years of work, the consultant team has not missed a single week of having one or more of its consultants at the hospital. . . .

[From I-C consultant's trip report, after two and

one-half years] ... Next came the afternoon seminar with all of the doctors.... Although this was my first day as a solo consultant [his previous trips had been with Chicago consultants], I was pleased with the response.... The doctors participated quite actively, and the time sped by quickly.... The group wished to continue the discussion next time.... All in all, it was a very satisfactory day; but I know that this might not have been the case were it not for the residual enthusiasm among the staff that was imparted by the Chicago team....

[Final Progress Report after three years] ... It has been a great experience for all of us on the consultant team, and in many ways we are sorry to see it end. There is also satisfaction and relief in finishing the job, however, and excitement at the prospect of our next state hospital project.

Enthusiasm for the project was clearly mutual. The consultants themselves found the project so stimulating and worthwhile that none of them dropped out and one member, Dr. Stewart, continued with the project even after moving to Cincinnati. The hospital staff, in turn, took pleasure and pride in the team's continuing enthusiastic interest in them. Those physicians who had suffered serious losses of self-esteem were especially buoyed by the consultants' acceptance of them as colleagues and confidence in what they could do — or, at least, could learn to do. Admittedly, the physicians were no doubt also influenced by certain tangible benefits they knew might accrue from successful participation in the training program — a certificate attesting to their training and the possibility of promotions.

Another contributing factor was the doctors' gradual-ly increasing sense of mastery of basic psychiatric knowl-edge and skills; they learned how to understand and deal with many difficult and disturbing problems of hospital-ized psychiatric patients. As their fears of mental illness and of the mentally ill lessened, their self-confidence cor-respondingly increased.

By the end of the second year, improvements in patient care and good therapeutic results with patients were beginning to feed back to the staff in the form of effects upon their morale. In the third year of the project, the unit teams noted healthy competition about thera-peutic results; and by that time, the development and stabilization of the interdisciplinary unit teams were contributing significantly to morale in the form of group support and the satisfactions of in-group membership.

Related to the subject of morale changes at the hospital was another effect of the project, this one extending beyond the hospital itself and into the com-munity of practicing psychiatrists. When, during its second year at the hospital, the consultant team contacted the psychiatrists in Illinois City and attempted to interest them in organizing a team of consultants which eventually would replace the commuting team,[1] the local psychi-atrists not only organized themselves as a consultant team to the state hospital; they worked along with the Chicago team for a year and then took over the project completely.

Prior to their joining together for purposes of this project, the local psychiatrists had had relatively little professional contact with each other; each had his own private practice and remained fairly isolated from his psychiatric colleagues. The consultant project brought

[1]See Chapter 8.

them together in a fruitful collaboration, one result of which was an effect upon their professional morale. The Chicago team coordinator reported:

> ... Dr. Stuckey invited me to come directly to his home from the airport to join the Illinois-City consultant team for their monthly planning meeting.... I was particularly impressed with the spirit and atmosphere of the I-C team's meeting, which had the same cooperative and candid tone that I believe characterizes the meetings of the Chicago team. The various members of the I-C team spoke up freely about their own ideas and their disagreements; matters were thrashed out in lively and constructive discussion, which moved gradually toward more or less general agreements about plans and policies. From my participation in this meeting, I feel all the more confident that the I-C consultants will be able to work together enjoyably and effectively as a smoothly functioning team....

The local consultant team formed a new professional organization, the Illinois City Neuropsychiatric Society, which the doctors at the state hospital were invited to join. The state hospital project provided the local psychiatrists with an opportunity to do some teaching, which they found stimulating and satisfying. Both the hospital staff and local consultants found their collaboration mutually rewarding.

Effects upon Professional Standards and Patient Care

By the end of the first year of the project, signs of improved professional standards were already apparent in the quality of case histories, psychological test reports, and social case studies. In addition were the clinical and research projects organized by the staff with the encouragement of the consultant team.

The Journal Club and the Education Committee were interdisciplinary in organization and membership—an early indication that departmental isolation eventually might be broken down. Collaboration with the Chicago team was also prominent in these developments, inasmuch as the consultants were asked to suggest articles for review by the Journal Club, and the coordinator of the consultant team was invited to participate in the monthly meetings of the Education Committee.

Still other indications of rising professional standards, increasing psychiatric knowledge and skills, and improved patient care became evident during the second year of the project: The doctors began to show greater interest in theoretical as well as practical clinical problems and started to do more psychiatric reading at that point. Some competition began to appear among the doctors for opportunities to attend a three-month special training program for state hospital physicians, held in Chicago at the Illinois State Psychiatric Institute. Dr. Bolley was one of the first to attend from Midwest. When the hospital was notified that Dr. Bolley had been the best trained in psychiatry of all the doctors participating in the ISPI program, the staff were extremely gratified and proud of their hospital, its doctors, and the consultant team. A marked increase in the admission rate of the hospital occurred during the second year of the project, as may be seen from a discussion of this development in the second-year progress report:

> The hospital staff and personnel deserve a great deal of credit for their patient and stead-

fast participation in our training programs. Our standards are high, and the training programs demanding. The staff's capacity for further training and higher skills is illustrated in various ways, one very tangible measure of which is the larger number of patients that they are now able to admit to the hospital and treat. The admission rate rose from 751 to 1,027 patients (per year) during the first two years of the project, and next year will be even higher. The rise in the admission rate has resulted from many more patients being transferred to Midwest State Hospital from metropolitan Chicago hospitals. Among other factors that may have contributed to the higher admission rate, we believe that the increasing professional skills and effectiveness of the hospital staff play an important part. (Concerning the latter conclusion, the consultant team had been told by state mental health officials that more patients were being transferred to Midwest Sate Hospital because the consultant team's project had produced a more active and effective therapeutic program at that hospital than was available in some of the seriously overcrowded and understaffed state hospitals in the vicinity of, and serving, metropolitan Chicago.)

The improvements in professional standards and patient care during the third year of the project began to be reflected more directly in humanistic concern for, and skillful professional attention to, the welfare and specific psychological needs of individual patients.[2] It may also

²These changes are reported more extensively in Chapter 7.

be of interest to note that during the third year of the project the discharge rate from the hospital rose from 73.3 per cent to 95.1 per cent, an increase of over twenty per cent.

Effects upon Interdisciplinary Functioning

Because the evolution toward team function has already been discussed, only a few words need be said here about this result of the project. The development of far-reaching and effective interdisciplinary functioning was a slowly evolving process and was not fully achieved until the unit system had been in effect for almost a year. Intense resistance to the unit system and the team approach characterized their early development. Disgruntled expressions of wanting to "go back to the old system, where we each had our own wards" were heard repeatedly; and the frictions between previously isolated staff members were so severe, at first, that the unit-team system almost certainly would have collapsed had it not been for the determination of the consultant teams to make the system work, and the weight of official support that it received from the administrative officers of the hospital.

After the new system had been established, however, one heard frequent expressions of, "How did we ever function without unit teams?"—a good question! In difficult and disturbing work such as that encountered in state hospitals, the adage that "two heads are better than one" is particularly appropriate. The personnel working in state hospitals need each others' mutual support, sharing of ideas, and cooperative carrying out of plans. Without such cooperation, individual efforts often conflict with each other or may even cancel each other out; and, worse still, everyone feels very much alone and more than a little frightened by the real, potential, and imagined dangers of the state hospital setting.

Another goal that may have been realized in part as a result of the unit system was an emphasis on a psychological approach to what are essentially psychological problems. Early in the development of the project, the consultants corresponded with Dr. Harry Wilmer of Palo Alto, who made a number of valuable suggestions about projected plans, goals, and methods. Wilmer raised the challenging question of who would be the "culture carriers" of the psychological approach after the team left the hospital. His question was answered partially by the local consultant team, which continued to emphasize the psychological approach, and partly by the unit teams, which supported and perpetuated this attitude — primarily through the opinions and suggestions of the psychologists, psychiatric social workers, and the activity therapists. These staff members knew *only* a psychological approach; they knew nothing about drugs or shock treatment. The doctors, and especially the Unit Chiefs, felt well enough trained in psychiatry and neurology to be fairly secure in their positions as leaders of the clinical teams. They had also become democratic enough to be able to let the voices of the nonmedical disciplines be heard in the team meetings.

Assuming that the foregoing impression is correct, the unit-team system takes credit for yet another important achievement. It seems that the most indelible mark left by the consultants on the hospital was an image, an image of a coordinated, effectively functioning, interdisciplinary team of professionals, all of whom were committed to and supported each other in a psychological approach to psychiatric problems. This lasting image at the hospital, in the form of the well-established, interdisciplinary unit teams, may be a significant part of the answer to Wilmer's question.

Effects upon the Consultant Team

In some respects, the consultant team changed as much in the years at Midwest as the hospital itself. Throughout the project, the team members experienced shifts in mood and morale — from the heights of exhilaration and excitement to the depths of discouragement and frustration. From both extremes, valuable lessons were learned.

A major source of dissatisfaction came with the realization of some undesirable features of the state hospital *system*. For example, the consultants were increasingly appalled at the demoralizing and dehumanizing effects of this system upon people, such as the herding of hundreds and hundreds of patients into huge, block-long dormitories, with beds huddled up one against the other in endless, depressing rows. The consultants not only had no intention of adjusting to these aspects of state hospital life, but resolved to change them in any way possible and with any measure available.

However, it was as necessary as it was painful to admit the limitations imposed by a system such as this one. There are things that simply cannot be done, changes that will not be made in state hospitals until the mores and concerns of the community dictate them. A state hospital is so much a political, economic, legal, and social reflection of its surroundings that it can alter only gradually and always in accord with the larger structure of which it is a part. This was a difficult reality for most of the team members to accept. But the lesson was learned, and the team came to measure its accomplishments on a different, more finely drawn scale than its members had ever used before, and to find satisfaction in small and simple achievements.

Changes also occurred in the team's teaching methods and content. The teachers learned to give special attention to problems of training motivation and resistance, and to proceed very slowly, stopping frequently to check whether they were being understood. The method of "relay teaching" (the same subject continued weekly by a series of consultant instructors) was introduced to increase the impact of certain seminars and to underscore certain fundamental concepts. Practical, demonstration types of teaching methods were used, including the "dynamimetic" interview (Fleming and Hamburg, 1958). In this method, the instructor usually acts the role of a patient, while a trainee interviews him (although the roles may be reversed). The interview is stopped, whenever necessary, to discuss technical and theoretical problems arising and then is resumed where it left off.

The consultants gradually came to recognize a need for almost endless repetition of courses in such basic skills as history-taking. This observation suggested that problems of retention of learning were not entirely solved by the approach of the Midwest project and that the limitations had to be compensated for by repetition of courses and by some provision for continued training at the hospital, in this case by the formation of the local teaching team from the Illinois-City area.

One final effect of the project upon the team was the development of an increased interest in broader aspects of mental health. Most of the team members also became more interested in trying to understand and treat patients with the severer forms of pathology—in their practices in

Chicago as well as in the state hospitals. From their work at Midwest, the consultants gained new hope about therapy with psychotic patients through the direct application of psychoanalysis, as well as the adaptation of psychoanalytic knowledge to other treatment techniques.

The effect of Midwest upon the consultants, therefore, was largely a broadening of outlook and interests, an opportunity for new applications of previous knowledge and skills and for new experiences in teamwork, multidisciplinary teaching, and state hospital psychiatry.

CHAPTER SEVEN

Improvements in Patient Care

WHILE CONSULTANTS HAVE ALL THE VULNERABILITIES of any "outsider," they also have the stranger's most powerful weapon, independence. At Midwest, as in all large and official institutions, procedures had altered over the years into rules, and the rules had solidified into "the way we do things." In such a situation, independent thought and action are apt to be considered the marks of the rebel, so that the innovator very soon departs, leaving the field to the cautious, the fearful, or the helpless—in this case, the career administrators, the doctors without training, and the patients.

The entire story of the consultant project at Midwest might be viewed as a frontal attack on the status quo of hospital life, a constant effort to push the policies aside to make room for the patients. To help them in this task, the consultants had more than specific technical knowledge; they had great freedom of ideas and action.

One of the stated major goals of the project had been "not primarily to increase the hospital discharge rate, but to raise the level of patient care for all patients, many of whom cannot be expected to leave the hospital ... the orientation of the project will be toward the individual patient." This statement was optimistic almost to the point of naïveté. Not only did the new team find a low ratio of medical staff to patients (about one to one hundred sixty), but the doctors were totally without psychiatric training. Such a combination spells standards of care that rarely can go beyond physical health and a clean shirt, and almost never into the realms of psychotherapy. This realization at first struck hard, as when a consultant reported on his initial visit:

> I was impressed by the readiness of the patients to reach out for contact, although in disguised and symbolic ways. The clinician in me, intrigued by this "Case material," was soon overwhelmed by the humanitarian side of my nature. It made me heartsick to think of how many of these patients, some of whom had given me hints that they could be "reached," were needlessly locked away in this hospital; at least they were not functioning as well as they might, even within the confines of the hospital.... I wonder whether we can really be effective in teaching here with the relatively dilute third-hand contact. I was appalled by the sordid atmosphere. The air [of this female ward] was foul-smelling and the room was filled with caricatures of human femininity.

All the consultants shared to some degree this initial feeling of being overwhelmed by needs that could not possibly be met by the resources at hand. But, even in the earliest days, there were some hopeful signs, responses of hospital personnel that might, with much careful nurturing, develop into therapeutic attitudes.

For example, it was striking to everyone how *something* seemed to happen in all cases where the consultants became involved with patients. Some patients improved "miraculously." This phenomenon is, of course, familiar to consultants everywhere; it is the remarkable response of a patient receiving concentrated individual attention for the first time. The value of such early demonstrations at Midwest lay less in the welfare of the patient than in an example to the staff: evidence that something *could* happen to a patient gave much-needed hope to the hospital personnel.

Some of the more dramatic of these events went beyond the group immediately concerned and became hospital landmarks, a part of the institution's history. The very first case handled by the consultants had such an impact on the staff. The patient was a thirteen-year-old boy seen by the psychiatric social work consultant on her second visit to the hospital. She reported:

The diagnosis made either at the clinic or the hospital sounded quite confusing, including such terms as "chronic brain syndrome." From the social worker's description, this did not sound like a psychotic child, though no one questioned his being in a mental hospital. It seemed to me that there was much confusion about planning. The hospital social worker really would have liked to work with the boy, but there was also some thought of transferring him to another state hospital . . . such a transfer would have removed him from all contact with his family. We decided that Dr. Simon should begin individual treatment with the boy, and one of the social workers with his mother. Since the child did not seem to need hospitalization, but was much disturbed by living with his mother, placement with the grandparents was arranged.

Soon afterward, the team coordinator's trip report mentioned the same case:

> The next conference was with Dr. Simon about the young boy he is treating. We met jointly with the social worker who is treating the boy's mother, and with Miss Jacob, who is her consultant. The joint conference was helpful to all of us. The patient has improved sufficiently that he has been conditionally discharged and is continuing to make progress on an out-patient basis. [A few months later, he reported again.] The patient is doing very well.... Simon is pleased with and proud of his work and is ready to start two more patients in supervised psychotherapy.

And, after reviewing this patient in a morning case conference, he added:

> There is no question that the staff were much impressed; you would have been delighted with Dr. Simon's pride when the conference was over.... I myself was not particularly modest about the gratifying outcome of this case, but wound up the seminar challenging the group somewhat dramatically: "*Now* do you see what can be done with psychotherapy, and with collaboration?" The group nodded thoughtfully and solemnly.

This case became locally famous for two reasons. It was the first attempt by the staff at providing treatment on an out-patient basis, thus making a more flexible use of hospital facilities than had previously been attempted. And it demonstrated the consultants' investment in individual patients, from diagnosis all the way through treatment and postdischarge follow-up.

The consultants repeatedly observed and reported on the effect of the team's constant concern with individuals.

> Everyone was impressed by the fact that this was the first time anyone has seen this young woman smile.

> One of the most striking developments in Dr. Christy since I have known him is the interest he now takes in individual patients. Formerly, he viewed his ward as a sort of undifferentiated mass of patients; he now knows each patient by name and by personal history. I think that's quite an accomplishment.

> Dr. Caine talked about a patient on his unit who has been viewed by aides as being combative. He believes that the patient is mentally retarded and that her behavior is not combative so much as a childlike, playful way of making contact. He is able to calm the patient by a firm and soothing approach. We talked about the importance of recognizing when such behavior is a form of making contact. In addition, we considered that with organic neurological deficits, the patient is likely to react to stimuli with a low threshold for frustration and possibly excitement. I advised him to explain the situation to the aides who work with the patient.

The final example combines a personal, human approach with some theoretical considerations; such concepts of human behavior gradually began to slip out of the classroom and into the wards and clinical discussions. The doctors and other personnel were learning, by observing, how a patient's words and actions make psychological "sense" and are the key to understanding and helping. The following is from one of the psychiatric social work consultant's trip reports:

> The rest of the morning was spent in the case conference; I interviewed the patient's mother for about an hour. Phil Seitz had interviewed the patient earlier. Although my interview was not as well focused as I would have liked, I felt I had succeeded in showing how, in an interview such as this, one can get a picture of a personality, her social surroundings, some of her history, as well as her characteristic manner of dealing with serious stresses . . . and the conflictful meaning that a specific child might have in a family constellation. I got the impression that the physicians were quite entranced with the material and with the mother. They were extremely quiet and attentive during the interview and, in the discussion period, asked very pertinent questions.

Another new departure for the hospital staff was the consultants' emphasis on improving the performance of all disciplines in order to improve the care of a single patient. Very early, there was a pinpointing of weaknesses in those departments with the greatest experience and the most training, the psychologists and social workers:

> The psychological report was based largely upon the conclusions from an interview, rather than

upon the psychological tests. I have the impression that their testing skills must have deteriorated to a considerable extent.

Social service had put together considerable information, but once again there had been no direct contact with the relatives except by phone.... The social workers need to be retrained in the importance of making and presenting the initial study of the patient as exhaustively as possible.

As soon as these deficiencies were noted, more emphasis was placed upon teaching conferences for the nonmedical departments, and the psychologists and social workers were included in all case discussions involving their departments—although the consultants limited this participation to the individuals personally concerned with the patient under discussion. The reports very soon began to take on a different flavor:

The case conference was unusually interesting ... the social history was gathered from four different individuals: the patient's husband, seventeen-year-old daughter, a state trooper who knows the family, and the family doctor who has cared for them for many years. All of this social history was well done and very helpful. For the first time, the work-up included a clear, personal impression of the personalities of the informants; I was glad the doctors had a chance to see how important the social worker's contribution can be.

The psychological report was excellent, and the psychologist, Mr. Martin, clearly had the most understanding of and interest in the patient. When I recommended individual rather than group therapy, the group agreed that Mr. Martin should be the therapist.

From this point on, the consultants began to note striking changes in the level of discussion during case conferences and heartening signs of a growing spirit of collaboration.

It should not be inferred that the hospital staff was totally immune to discouragement or a slackening of its new-found therapeutic attitudes. The following examples of such periods of discouragement are only two of many:

> The doctor thought that, since the patient had relapsed, we would now give up our work with him and forget about the case. I explained to him that this was simply one episode in the course of the patient's treatment and, although it might cause us to modify our treatment plan, we would go on working with the patient together.

> Dr. Christy continues to follow his old medical attitude of focusing upon improvement in the symptoms, instead of adopting a somewhat more passive and patient attitude of simply trying to understand what is going on. Each time the patient shows a fresh wave of delusions, Dr. Christy becomes discouraged and is ready to quit. I am trying to help him develop a more inquiring curiosity about each such episode in the course of the patient's psychosis, and also to emphasize some of the positive (e.g. restitutive) aspects of the delusions.

Sometimes the goals were set too high, and then it became the task of the consultants to puncture unrealistic balloons. The psychology consultant confronted the entire group of staff psychologists with the dilemma they had created for themselves by maintaining inappropriate therapeutic goals:

> This led to an interesting but somewhat painful discussion about issues of morale, staff esteem, and sources of satisfaction. It was like a session in group therapy. Certainly, no solutions came of it, but some of the feelings, some of their expectations of themselves and their tendencies to blame the patient for therapeutic "failure" became very clear. I talked with one psychologist afterward, and we both had the feeling that this group did not use one potential source of satisfaction, i.e., the satisfaction of intellectual curiosity. Instead, they think only of the impossible therapeutic goal of "complete cure" and are inclined to see the therapist as the potent contributor to either success or failure.

The consultants, too, had episodes of discouragement directly related to hopes for a patient's welfare. It was a new experience for most of the Chicagoans, whose professional lives had few legal overtones, to be faced with the restrictions of state institutions. There was, for instance, the law that requires patients to be transported back to their states of residence for commitment unless some special financial arrangement can be worked out. In one case, such arrangements proved impossible, and a patient with deep roots in the Illinois-City area had to be sent to her own state, a thousand miles away. Such occurrences, flying in the face of everyone's professional judgment and therapeutic hopes, made the consultants as angry as they did the hospital personnel. On the other hand, some episodes evoking righteous indignation had good results. On a trip to a ward of very regressed women patients, the psychiatric social work consultant found an extremely angry aide. Pressed for reasons, she said that the movies shown on her ward twice each week had been discontinued as not being worthwhile. The aide knew that many of her "ladies" did not pay attention to the movies, but, "Some of them did, and for them it meant something; they get little enough on this ward!" The aide's willingness to fight for her "ladies" was impressive, and support from the social work staff and consultant led to a reinstatement of the movies and to a new conviction on the part of the aide that her battle for her patients was worth waging.

Despite many improvements, punitive attitudes toward the patients continued to appear for a long time. Not until as late as the third year of the project did the hospital staff discontinue an initial diagnostic evaluation conference for new patients, which the consultants had criticized earlier as "brutal" to the patients. These conferences were arranged in compliance with a well-meaning but misguided state regulation requiring that ι diagnosis and treatment plan be established and entered in the chart of every patient within forty-eight hours after admission to the hospital—far too early to make such clinical decisions in many cases, or to have obtained sufficient information about the patient on which to base such decisions. When the consultants began attending these meetings, they were so appalled at the way the conferences were conducted, they felt the only suggestion they could make was that the conferences be discontinued. The following excerpts from selected trip reports during that period give an indication of what distressed them:

... I sat in on the Intake Conference for the first time. I kept my own participation in the conference to a minimum and acted more as an observer. . . . I was struck by the physical arrangement of the room and afterward felt I must suggest that this be changed. The doctor was seated at an oversized library-type table in front of the large staff group, the latter sitting in rows of chairs facing the table. The patient was brought in and seated beside the doctor at the front table, facing the group. While both doctor and patient sat facing the large "audience," without facing or looking at each other, the doctor "interrogated" the patient. A secretary sat at one end of the big table, writing down everything that was said, disconcertingly like a court reporter. It seemed terribly artificial and depressingly reminiscent of a courtroom. When I mentioned this to the doctors afterward, they said: "This is the way it is always done." I suggested that the setting and procedure of the conference be changed: that they get rid of the table and the secretary and the courtroom atmosphere; that the doctor sit facing the patient and be more considerate of the patient's feelings, his anxiety and embarrassment; that the doctor try to establish some rapport with the patient, rather than start out so abruptly with matter-of-fact "interrogation." I don't know whether the suggestions will do any good. . . .

The same psychiatric consultant, a month later:

... In the morning I went to the Intake Conference again. . . . Necessary as these conferences may be, it seems to me that they are a tremendous waste of time, in addition to being inhumane and a potential danger to the patients. The "evaluations" are made on the basis of very inadequate information—a few extra days to find out more about the patient would make the same amount of time much more humanely and effectively spent. The danger is that labels are put on the chart at this time which follow the patient through the rest of his hospitalization, and which become the basis for all future planning. Having once "categorized" the patient, the doctor is then free to go on his way. In other words, there is a premature closure. What shall we do about this deplorable situation?...

Team coordinator, the following month:

... I attended the Intake Conference, and, so help me, I don't believe *anyone* knew what was going on there. There must be a lot of nonverbal communication that goes on in these dreadful meetings, because somehow they got the patient "staffed" and the ritual note dictated to the secretary. I told Dr. Simon [the new Acting Clinical Director] how appalled the consultants are at these meetings and added that we feel they should be discontinued. To my surprise, he agreed....

It took a long time, however—more than a year—before these intake meetings were finally abolished. They were eventually replaced by clinical conferences of the unit teams.

The unit-team system was the final and perhaps most

effective step in focusing the attention of the hospital personnel upon the individual patient. With the introduction of this system, the doctors began to take more and more responsibility for the improvement of patient care. An example:

> Dr. Bolley said that his team had come to the conclusion that new patients admitted to their unit should be kept and treated at the Admissions Building if at all possible, rather than transferring them after a short trial of intensive treatment to the more chronic wards. In the old days, he said, the doctors who worked at the Admissions Building were so overburdened with working up new patients that they often transferred them to chronic wards, where they would be under the care of other doctors. His team has come to realize that if a patient is sent to a chronic ward, the patient tends to *become* chronic. Their present policy, therefore, is to transfer patients from their admitting wards to out-lying wards only as an absolute last resort. Dr. Bolley believes this is one of the reasons their discharge rate has gone up so dramatically in the past six months. Among other reasons suggested to explain the success of this new policy and procedure was the interesting observation that the relatives of patients begin to reduce their visits to the patient drastically when the patient is transferred to a chronic, dilapidated, and, in some respects, disgraceful back ward. As long as the patient remains in the active-treatment part of the hospital, the relatives tend to maintain their interest in him and hope for his recovery. . . .

Patient resonsibility now becomes a closely, sometimes jealously guarded matter:

> ...Drs. Christy and Willens said that the prob-
> lems they have now are not so much within the
> unit team itself, which is functioning smoothly
> and cooperatively, but with the "Top Chiefs."
> They explained that occasionally the Top Chiefs
> will make decisions about certain patients that
> the unit team feels to be matters for the team
> itself to decide. "We consider all plans and
> decisions about our patients to be unit prob-
> lems," Christy said firmly. I was impressed with
> this attitude and comment—partly because it
> expresses so emphatically the cohesive and col-
> laborative feeling of the unit team as a unified
> group, but also partly because in the old days the
> doctors were not at all jealous of their right to
> make decisions and plans concerning patients.
> In the past, they often tried to get us, or the Top
> Chiefs, or *someone* to take the responsibility for
> clinical decisions. I believe that the doctors' new
> attitude of confidence and firmness about their
> right and wish to make such decisions themselves
> comes from two main developments: one is the
> fact that they know a good deal more about
> clinical psychiatry now, i.e., have more clinical
> skill and confidence; but another reason must be
> that they are obtaining a considerable amount of
> support and security from the collaboration of
> teammates within their unit teams....

By the time the Midwest project terminated for the
Chicago team, the attitudes toward patients and the

quality of care that patients were receiving had undergone significant changes—the stability and permanence of which, however, had yet to be tested. Although the hospital was handling more patients than ever before, the focus was now set upon the diagnosis and plan of treatment for each individual and shared responsibility by a small group for his well-being. Undoubtedly, many factors contributed to the development and continuation of this new trend in patient care.

One such factor was probably that the consultants maintained consistently high standards throughout the project. Another was the presence of the local Illinois-City consultant team, whose members were psychiatrists with a dedication to psychotherapeutic work with individual patients. Still another factor was the stimulation provided by regular therapeutic contacts with patients and the personal gratifications that come from such work. By the time the consultants left the hospital, there was reason to hope that this upward trend in patient care would continue.

CHAPTER EIGHT

The Illinois-City Consultant Team

ALMOST FROM THE BEGINNING of its identity as a team, the Chicago group had in mind it own eventual replacement at Midwest. No matter what might be accomplished at the hospital in the experimental three years, it would have been little short of miraculous had the improvements held without further reinforcement during the years ahead. Most to be feared, of course, was the regressive pull to the old and familiar routines when the new, often challenging, and always watchful consultants withdrew. It therefore seemed evident to the consultants and to the Midwest staff that plans must be made for continued teaching at the hospital.

Just as clear as the need for a replacement team was the necessity for recruiting it from the neighborhood of the hospital, inasmuch as neither the airplane nor boundless goodwill could make a permanent commuting team from Chicago feasible. It seemed only logical to look around the immediate Illinois-City area for psychiatrists and other professional consultants to replace the Chicagoans at Midwest.

Toward the end of the second year, the nucleus of an Illinois-City consultant team was formed. Attracted largely by the teaching opportunities at the hospital, four psychiatrists and a neurosurgeon responded to the first feelers put out by the Chicago team. It was agreed jointly that the new team should get its Midwest introduction by accompanying the Chicago consultants on their visits, observing and participating increasingly in the various teaching activities. Late in the second year of the project, Dr. Stuckey of the newly formed team made his first visit to the hospital, and the Chicago team coordinator reported:

> I have the impression that Dr. Stuckey's approach to patients and problems is very similar to our own, i.e., an approach that is at once human and dynamic. I am more hopeful than ever that he will become the coordinator of a local consultant team. Another factor which I believe is in favor of his being the one for that role is the fact that he and the Superintendent seem to get along so well together, understand each other, and speak the same language about patients.

The initial phase of the program was pursued for six months, followed by another six months in which the I-C team gradually took over the project. During the latter period, the Chicago consultants accompanied their I-C counterparts to the hospital only once a month. This plan permitted a gradual pull-out by the Chicago team and a gradual transition to take-over by the I-C team. By the end of their three years of commuting to Midwest, the Chicago team had discontinued its trips and the Illinois-City group was completely independent and in charge of the project—meeting with the Unit Chiefs, moderating the conferences and seminars, and, within a few more months, becoming involved in special research projects as well.

The new team members differed from each other both in background and in approach to clinical and teaching problems. Three had a good deal of previous experience in state hospitals; two had never set foot in such an institution before. But they soon demonstrated a commitment to the project and to each other as an interdisciplinary teaching team. From their earliest group meetings, they adopted their predecessors' system of regular reports following each tour of duty at the hospital; their reports present a development so similar to that of the Chicago group as to be almost a mirror reflection of the earlier experience, suggesting that the process had a momentum all its own.

The Illinois-City consultants began at the same high level of optimism as the Chicago team and, like them, suffered through periods of discouragement and frustration. Much of the disappointment touched on familiar questions of staff training and motivation for further learning. The new team, too expressed dissatisfaction with the doctors' history-taking skills, their level of sophistication, and their performance in therapeutic work with patients. They soon came to feel that the existence of the physicians' Journal Club depended less on the enthusiasm of its own members than upon the initiative of the consultants. And, for a period of many months, the new consultants felt that they had only paper acceptance in the administrative quarters of the hospital. In support of this feeling, they could point to one small incident and to another more threatening event. Unimportantly, but perhaps significantly, none of the new consultants was invited to the staff Christmas party at the hospital during the first year of work there. And only weeks after they began their regular visits, the Superintendent imported an autonomous group of psychology consultants from another city, a move he made without collaborating with the I-C team. Although later familiarity and a common goal helped to heal this two-team wound, the area remained a bit sore under the surface for rather a long time.

As might be expected, there were administrative complaints to match those of the consultants, and these anxieties soon took the form of a demand to receive copies of all consultant team reports and communications.

Faced with a prickly handful of problems, the I-C team requested a meeting with the Chicago team to review the situation. In general, it was the Chicago group's impression that the I-C consultants had developed a fairly comfortable and effective working alliance and were successfully maintaining the professional standards recently set at Midwest. Participation in their training seminars was fairly active, the unit-team system had held together, and the medical, psychological, and social work departments had all recently added new personnel who were working competently on the wards. The over-all hospital picture was also very good, with an all-time high rate of discharge coupled with an all-time low patient census.

Nevertheless, the irritations and frustrations felt by the I-C team were real enough. They were similar in kind and degree to the feelings of the Chicago team three years before and were probably inevitable "growth pangs" that would accompany any such new attempt. But it seemed also that a part of the team's disappointment arose from its own elevated expectations. The new group had reasoned that, since the Chicago team had been able to train the staff to a point of fairly adequate knowledge and skill, they themselves should take up from that point and speed full steam ahead, almost without limit or loss of pace. Each step back or hesitation thus carried more than its due share of discouragement. The group was ready to agree that its sights had been set unrealistically and that it might better set goals that would allow for a gradual upward movement without either steep rises or very sharp falls.

The most important result of this special meeting with the Chicago team was the agreement to set up a collaborative re-evaluation and planning meeting with the hospital administration and staff. Within a month, such a conference was arranged and proved, in retrospect, to be a turning point in hospital-consultant team relationships and communication.[1]

At this all-day session, the entire educational program was discussed in great detail, with particular stress placed on clarifying the relationship of the teaching team to the hospital staff and administration. The consultants clearly stated their primary aim to be the teaching of the staff, and they agreed to requests from the staff for a more tightly structured curriculum. Although they were unable at this time to secure the personal involvement of the hospital administrators in either the teaching or clinical programs, it was agreed that there should be a four-man coordinating committee consisting of an I-C team member, an administrative officer, one of the psychology consultants, and a member of the hospital staff. This brain-child was happily conceived, but died aborning; the plan for a coordinating committee never materialized.

[1] So successful was this meeting, that such conferences became a regular feature of the Chicago team's second state hospital project.

Two other developments associated with the joint re-evaluation and planning meeting also appeared to be important. One was that the hospital administration apologized to the consultant team for lack of collaboration with them about the addition of psychology consultants from another city. This made it quite clear that the administrators definitely wanted to keep the I-C team and were willing to extend themselves in its behalf. The Superintendent's willingness to make amends in this matter took considerable courage and character; this single act may well have saved the I-C team's relationship with the hospital.

The other development at this time was an agreement among the I-C consultants to rotate the time-consuming and often tedious job of team coordinator. The change-over to a new coordinator was smooth and may have constituted a milestone in the I-C consultants' relations with each other as a team. Their agreement to share an important leadership function may have helped to bring them closer to each other and may also have helped to relieve competitive pressure within the group; for shortly after these developments, the I-C team instituted "relay teaching" for the first time and agreed firmly to carry on the regular trip reports, which, for reasons shortly to be described, they had considered discontinuing.

Following the joint re-evalution and planning meeting, the reports from the I-C team began to take on a tone of greater optimism and satisfaction. Within a month of the meeting, an I-C consultant stated his impression that the hospital administrators "now seemed to be extremely anxious that we are all pleased by our reception and they are trying hard to make sure that everything we might need is available to us." He added: "I feel we have a going

project here and that it will continue to operate." Signs of
concurrence in this optimism were evident among the
medical staff. The doctors began dropping in on each
other's supervisory conferences, requesting seminars on
special topics, and generally responding with an enthusiasm that an I-C team member described as "infectious
and productive." As the doctors became more and more
involved in decisions about the planning of their own
curricula, they became increasingly free with their
teachers, candidly expressing criticisms of the consultants'
teaching techniques. Because such complaints were acted
upon promptly, the communication between the two
groups continued to improve with each visit. The Unit
Chiefs also felt free enough to mention at this point
that they would like to have more contact with the I-C
consultants outside the hospital.

A series of changes in teaching style and content were
introduced by the I-C team, for the most part aimed at
combating inertia and resistance to the training program.
Within the next six months, there was a gradual but
definite shift away from formal didactic instruction toward a group-centered type of seminar, which encouraged
the participants to think for themselves and to participate
in decisions about their own training needs. By the end of
their first year, some of the I-C consultants were even
encouraging the doctors to moderate the teaching case
conferences, with the consultant sitting in as resource
person.

Another change in teaching method was the introduction of "relay teaching," which had been used with
such success by the Chicago team, wherein each consultant
continued a subject where the teacher of the previous week
left it. This system made it possible to concentrate on one

subject at a time and to achieve greater frequency, continuity, and impact in certain training seminars. The I-C consultants grew to like the system and were pleased with its results. Occasionally, the method broke down, as when trip reports arrived too late for the next teacher's use.

The subject matter of the seminars also underwent alteration. Increasingly, the consultants veered away from their earlier emphasis on diagnosis, symptom patterns, and psychopharmacology to a new stress on psychiatric histories, psychodynamics, and psychotherapy.

All these changes were brought about quite gradually, as can be illustrated by three examples:

The first was a change in the attitude of one of the I-C team teachers toward the hospital doctors, as reflected by his choice of words, in his reports, to describe his approach in teaching them. At the beginning of the first year he spoke of "gentle persuasion"; in subsequent memos he was "chiding" them, was a "gadfly" "hammering away at basic concepts," and, finally, "pounding."

Another example occurred in connection with the doctors' seminar on psychiatric history-taking and examination. Despite complaints by the doctors that they were tired of studying this subject, the I-C consultants insisted that the training be continued until the physicians had better mastery of these basic skills. Persistence in this area eventually paid off.

The third example of firmness occurred toward the end of the first year, when statements began to appear in the I-C trip reports that the consultants were reporting to the Superintendent clinical and training deficiencies among certain staff members, seeking his help in "getting the staff to work and study harder." This method of using the Superintendent's power and authority as leverage produced quick but only temporary results. It was, frankly, a mistake, as the consultants quickly discovered, for it threatened to disrupt rapport between consultants and staff.

As the medical program became more effective, the nonmedical departments began to seek help from the consultants, first making their interest known by attending the medical conferences as uninvited guests. The I-C team took the hint and responded by establishing special training programs for four other disciplines: the social workers, activity therapists, nurses, and volunteers. In addition, the psychology consultants from a nearby city and a new psychiatric social worker were integrated with the I-C team and served as consultants to their respective departments.

With increasing success in their teaching, the I-C team found new gratification from and motivation for the project. Their primary motivation had been their interest in teaching, a goal that was now being reached and satisfied. One of the I-C consultants reported that he continued "to be amazed and pleased at the enthusiasm and interest of the Activity Therapy Staff." Another consultant reported that his new seminars with the psychiatric social work staff were "going exceedingly well." With somewhat less enthusiasm, a third consultant commented that the nurses, who had been the most resistant to training, were "becoming somewhat less catatonic" in their seminars. He mentioned in the same report that he was "gratified to find that the doctors are extremely interested in attempting to understand underlying dynamics of the cases." He also reported favorably on a new training method he had instituted in group therapy, in which selected doctors came to his clinic to observe his work with therapy groups. A statement by still another I-C consultant clearly expressed the improved morale and outlook of the I-C team:

> At the end of the afternoon, I left Midwest State Hospital in a considerably better frame of mind than the one with which I had arrived. The weather was dismal, I was behind schedule, and my arrival was delayed by not one, but two freight trains at the crossing. My mood improved steadily throughout the afternoon by virtue of the very active response of the doctors to the afternoon's activities.

The feeling between the I-C team and the hospital administration also became more cordial following the joint re-evaluation and planning conference, although the regular weekly contacts of the various consultants with the Superintendent, Assistant Superintendent, and Clinical Director continued to be rather shallow — "passing the time with pleasantries," rather than digging into the innumerable training and related clinical problems facing them. The Chicago team had had similar difficulties in establishing a candid, genuine, and productive rapport with the administration. An I-C consultant observed that "the relationship with the administration seems more relaxed and natural now." Another consultant's report of the I-C team meeting that month mentioned that "conflicts with the hospital administration are now mostly minor skirmishes."

But indications of deeper difficulties between the hospital administration and consultant team became evident whenever the consultants made recommendations concerning administrative policies and procedures at the hospital. The hospital administrators often reacted to such suggestions defensively, as though their prerogatives were being threatened. It appeared that the administration would have preferred that the consultant team confine itself strictly to teaching. Some of the I-C consultants insisted, however, that it was part of their function to advise the administration on hospital policies and practices that might either improve the clinical, teaching, and research programs or facilitate changes in those existing policies and practices they found to be antitherapeutic, antieducational, or unscientific.

An example of this problem was reported by an I-C consultant who discovered on certain wards an antitherapeutic practice of which the administration was not aware. "The attendants make the patients go to bed at 6:00 P.M. so they can clean up the wards for the night."

A strong statement about this issue had been made by the original I-C team coordinator at the joint evaluation and planning meeting:

> I feel that the consultants should be available not only as teachers giving lectures and consultations, but also to the administration and to everybody else in discussing certain aspects of the hospital routines, or anything else that is pertinent to the treatment and handling of patients. I am not interested in how the administration hires personnel, how they report admissions and discharges, or anything else that pertains to purely administrative matters; but I do feel definitely that it is within the domain of the consultants to make suggestions from time to time that might improve the situation and condition of patients and the treatment opportunities that are available.

There were other indications of friction between the top administration and the consultant team. A fairly serious crisis developed when the administration, feeling troubled by the I-C team's confidential reports to each other, requested that they (the administration) receive copies of these reports. After considering the possibility of discontinuing the trip reports, the I-C team members eventually decided to hold firm on their right and need to have private communication with each other. The administration gave in on this issue.

Later on, the I-C team coordinator learned that, at the Chicago team's new project at a second state hospital, the Superintendent had turned over to a Senior Staff Committee the power to make decisions about all matters pertaining to the consultant team's teaching programs—an administrative arrangement that had worked out exceedingly well. The I-C team coordinator described this to the Superintendent at Midwest, but he was definitely opposed to such a plan, which he felt would be designed primarily to take over his power and authority.

Despite the surface amenities between the hospital administration and I-C team, therefore, deeper sources of disturbance, conflict, and strain were apparent. How to improve this problem is a moot question; but its answer is probably contingent upon a candid, honest, mutually respecting and continually developing relation between the hospital administration and the members (especially the coordinator) of the consultant team.

A word may be said at this point about the I-C team's teaching and supervision of the unit teams. It had been agreed at the time of the change-over to the I-C team that the new consultants should be both the "watch dogs" of the unit system—seeing to it that the unit teams were not

allowed to fragment or become simply "paper organizations"—and the training consultants to these important
functional groups, helping them to continue developing
themselves both in their clinical skills and as teams. The
I-C consultants pursued this goal through regular conferences with the Unit Chiefs and teaching case conferences
with the unit teams. The unit system was so well maintained by the hospital administration, staff, and I-C team
that it was used as a model by the Chicago consultants'
second state hospital, for the organization and development of its own unit system.

As noted earlier, there were many parallels in the
development and evolution of the I-C and Chicago teams.
During the first few months at Midwest, the consultants
became acquainted with the staff and gradually developed
the initial training curricula and schedules. During that
period, the consultants' time at the hospital was taken up
almost exclusively with staff members rather than with
patients. As this phase of the project drew to a close, the
consultants began to spend more time going to the wards
with the staff to see patients.

After an initial period of discouragement about the
educability of the staff, the consultants began to observe
indications of progress in the hospital personnel, which
rekindled their hopes. The consultants gradually "jelled"
as a team during these initial phases of the projects, in the
course of which they tended to develop a certain proprie-
tary feeling that *all* educational matters at the hospital were
the province of the consultant team. Two different Superintendents then challenged this prerogative of the consultant
teams by bringing in other training consultants. The I-C
team reacted to the Superintendent's abrupt introduction
of psychology consultants in much the same way that the

Chicago team reacted to the previous Superintendent's unannounced decision to send staff physicians to a local college for a course in psychology.

Next, a phase of staff resistance to the training program set in. This seemed to occur when the staff began to see more clearly how much work and study the training program would require. The consultant teams handled this problem by use of special clinical and research projects and by a shift toward more group-centered and collaborative teaching methods. These changes carried the training programs through to their more definitive conclusions.

Despite the problems faced by the I-C team, the hospital staff, and the administration in their work together, the progress they made was impressive. The relationship between hospital and consultant team, though not all they would have liked it to be, endured, deepened, and improved. The I-C consultants held together as a team and carried the responsibility of the project on their own for four more years, after the Chicago consultants had completed their teaching at Midwest. The I-C team earned the distinction therefore, of being the first[2] team of consultants to have combined and coordinated their efforts successfully in support of a large, public mental hospital in their own community. That the I-C team eventually disbanded after half-a-dozen years of working together should give cause for neither regret nor criticism. By the time it discontinued, the hospital staff had taken over and were conducting the necessary training programs themselves—which, perhaps more than anything else, strengthens our confidence in the consultant-team approach.

[2]A somewhat similar project was attempted on a smaller scale by a group of psychiatrists in the community of another Illinois state hospital some years ago, but the effort failed, owing to lack of coordination and follow-through.

Appendix

A Review of the Literature
on State Hospital Psychiatry

A REVIEW OF THE REFERENCES to the literature[1] on state hospital psychiatry resulted in a somewhat surprising discovery. The literature falls naturally into three principal sets of *Problems,* on the one hand, and three principal sets of *Trends and Improvements,* on the other.

I. Problems
   A. Largeness and isolation
   B. State hospital organization and functioning
      1. Social systems aspects and studies
      2. Monolithic, authoritarian administrative structure
      3. Interdisciplinary communication and collaboration
   C. Patient care and treatment
      1. Manpower shortages—in both numbers and skills of staff
      2. Weakness of clinical leadership
      3. Custodial in contrast to therapeutic patient care
II. Trends and Improvements
   A. Decentralization and teamwork
      1. The unit system

[1]The actual references have been assembled and indexed by subject matter (see p. 237).

    2. Interdisciplinary clinical teams
    3. Fuller use of ancillary personnel
B. Social psychiatric approaches
    1. Group, milieu, and therapeutic community methods
    2. Open *vs.* closed wards and hospitals
    3. Increased participation and self-regulation by patients in therapeutic programs and ward government
    4. Participation of families in therapeutic planning and rehabilitation
    5. Partial hospitalization, follow-up, and after care
    6. Community resources and liaison; community psychiatry
C. Training and research
    1. Training programs—for improved professional skills in individual disciplines and also in interdisciplinary collaboration
    2. Research programs
    3. The consultant team approach

The foregoing sequence of problems, trends, and improvements expresses roughly the amount of attention that has been paid to these topics investigatively over the past ten to twenty years.[2] Investigations and reports during this period have emphasized the social-systems aspects and administrative characteristics of state hospitals, at the same time stressing social psychiatric approaches to problems of patient care and treatment. Administrative decentralization of state hospitals into autonomous units staffed by interdisciplinary clinical teams is a growing trend. The training and research needs of state hospitals have received the least attention.

[2]See the attached Bibliography and Subject Index.

Problems of Largeness and Isolation

The problem of largeness of state hospitals received its most forceful acknowledgment when the Final Report of the Joint Commission on Mental Illness and Health, *Action for Mental Health* (1961), recommended unequivocally that no psychiatric hospital of the future should have more than one thousands beds. Most state hospitals have several times that number. Numerous surveys and critiques of state mental hospitals have agreed that these institutional behemoths are far too large for personalized, humanistic care and treatment of individual patients. The largeness of such institutions appears to contribute also to many if not all of the major problems of state hospital psychiatry: the monolithic, administrative structure of such institutions, difficulties in interdisciplinary communication and collaboration, manpower shortages, weakness of clinical leadership, and custodial in contrast to therapeutic patient care.

In addition to the oppressive effects upon the morale of the people who live and work in these huge, relatively isolated institutions, the remoteness from metropolitan centers also reduces the opportunities of the staff for additional training. As a result, patient care suffers, the staff feels even more frustrated and discouraged, morale sinks lower, many staff members leave the hospital, the constant turnover of staff disrupts continuity of patient care — all of which contributes to custodial in contrast to therapeutic care of patients in such hospitals.

Various methods have been developed to reduce the problems of largeness and isolation in state mental hospitals. One of the most promising of such trends is the administrative decentralization of such hospitals into autonomous units staffed by interdisciplinary clinical teams of psychiatrists, psychologists, psychiatric social workers, psychiatric nurses, activities therapists, psychiatric aides, volunteers, chaplains, and others. In effect, the formation of such units divides a single, oversized mental institution into several smaller hospitals, each with a more reasonable and workable number of patients — usually considerably less than a thousand. Also characteristic of the unit system are the policies and practices of "progressive hospitalization" and "continuous patient care" — i.e., each unit has facilities for all types of patients and all phases of hospitalization, so that a patient admitted to a particular unit always remains the patient of the same clinical team, rather than being shifted from one group of hospital personnel to another whenever ward transfers are made.

The unit system entails a type of decentralized organization within large state hospitals that approximates the management and staffing patterns of smaller hospitals. In addition to the improvements brought about in direct clinical services to patients, the unit plan also facilitates more efficient and effective ongoing, in-service, staff training programs for all hospital personnel. The reason for the latter advantage is that the unit team becomes a convenient and natural locus, not only for clinical and administrative decisions concerning patients, but also for staff training activities. Whether in-service training is the responsibility of an educator group within the hospital or from the "outside," with the institution of a unit system many hospital training activities become increasingly interdisciplinary, rather than divided exclusively along disciplinary lines, and tend to be carried out within the individual unit teams.

By far the majority of reports on the unit plan indicate that this system provides considerably improved patient care. The principal drawbacks of the unit plan are problems of administration and staffing.

With respect to interdisciplinary clinical teams, which constitute the staffs of the decentralized, autonomous units, *in-patient* teams are still relatively uncommon. Most such clinical teams in psychiatry have been developed in out-patient settings. One of the several important advantages of such teams in remotely located state hospitals is a reduction of the sense of professional isolation which can be so oppressive to staff members in these institutions.

The literature on psychiatric teams suggests that effective team functioning requires considerable competence of each team member in at least three important respects: (1) each member of the team must have achieved considerable mastery of the subject matter and the professional skills of his own particular discipline; (2) he must have acquired practical experience and skills in collaborative working together with heterogeneous groups; and (3) he needs to have reached a state of personal and professional security enabling him to accept a viewpoint about group functioning in which leadership is considered a function shared by all members of the team rather than the prerogative or responsibility of any one person.

Another trend that has improved the problems of largeness and isolation in state hospitals is the development of social psychiatric approaches. This collaborative joining of all available forces—including those of the patients themselves—in the service of better care and treatment of the mentally ill has made it more possible to reach the large masses of patients in the state hospitals by group, milieu, and therapeutic community methods. It has also reduced the isolation of these institutions in a number of other ways by promoting open wards and hospitals, encouraging greater participation of families in therapeutic planning and rehabilitation, increasing participation and self-regulation by patients in therapeutic programs and ward government, establishing facilities and procedures for partial hospitalization, follow-up, and aftercare, and by increased liaison with community agencies. Concerning the relationship of state hospitals and community resources, some writers have recommended that state hospitals become the "cornerstones of community mental health services," "community mental health centers," and "educational and social agencies for the community." Others have questioned whether goals of this kind for state hospitals can be realized, since—among other limitations—these institutions are not usually located in centers of population density.

Problems of State Hospital Organization and Administration

In past years, many articles dealt with some of the administrative and organizational features, problems, and peculiarities of large isolated state mental hospitals. For the most part, these studies were carried out by social scientists who investigated various social-systems aspects of the organization and functioning of state hospitals. As is well known, the traditional administrative and power structure of these venerable institutions is authoritarian and monolithic. One of the several factors appearing to promote this type of organizational structure is fear— some real, some imaginary—about the potentially dangerous and chaotic situation in institutions that were once called "lunatic asylums." Other contributing factors include the largeness and isolation of these institutions, manpower shortages — particularly, a relative lack of highly skilled professional personnel — social and political pressures, etc.

One of the consequences of a monolithic administrative structure is that its members direct much of their attention, interest, and communications toward the authority-figure at the top of the hierarchy. As a result, lateral communication among persons on the same administrative level, and even communication with subordinates, may be constricted and diminished. Rivalry with peer personnel for the favor of the authority-figure may be intensified. In some instances, the person in authority may use and manipulate this rivalry to keep subordinates divided and loyal only to himself, rather than banded together cooperatively. These tendencies militate against interdisciplinary, interdepartmental communication and collaboration. Instead, one often finds among the various departments a chronic, destructive suspiciousness of and spying upon each other, sporadic outbursts of internecine warfare, long-standing interpersonal and intergroup vendettas, extremely poor — or even no — communication between disciplines, and relatively little clinical cooperation for the benefit of patients. In addition, as a number of investigators have shown, these conflicts and tensions among the hospital staff are frequently reflected in the symptom fluctuations of patients.

One of the administrative trends that may offer substantial improvement over the older, monolithic tradition in state mental institutions is decentralization, with the formation of autonomous units staffed by interdisciplinary clinical teams. Still another trend that may help to improve these problems is the upsurge of research into the social-systems aspects of large mental institutions. The very process of such a hospital studying itself—of allowing itself to be studied—appears to set the stage for and to initiate a process of change in the institution.

Social-systems studies are intimately related to another growing general trend in state hospitals, that of social psychiatric approaches to problems of patient care and treatment. This trend toward collaborative teamwork may be seen in virtually all branches and aspects of state hospital psychiatry: in the unit systems of certain hospitals; in the development of interdisciplinary psychiatric teams; the attention paid to group-process problems of people working together; fuller use of ancillary personnel; increasing participation of patients themselves in their own treatment and self-regulation; patient government; ward-milieu and therapeutic-community methods; the integration of men and women patients on psychiatric wards; other sciences, becoming involved in the widening fields of social psychiatry; racial desegregation within hospitals; participation of families in therapeutic planning and rehabilitation; teamwork among consultants to psychiatric institutions—described in the body of this book; collaboration among various psychiatric institutions; assorted forms of partial hospitalization; the community mental health center concept; integration of hospital and community resources. Still other trends that may help to bring about improvements in the problems of state hospital organization and administration are training and research programs (discussed in the next section).

Problems of Patient Care and Treatment

The principal problem of patient care and treatment in many state hospitals is the tendency to provide custodial care rather than active, sophisticated, and effective *treatment* for patients. All of the problems of state hospital psychiatry discussed previously contribute to this tendency, i.e., the large numbers of patients; the relative isolation of patients and staff; manpower shortages, both in numbers and skills of the staff; a monolithic administrative structure which tends to stifle rather than facilitate interdisciplinary teamwork and creative coping with problems; and insufficient use of ancillary personnel, including patients themselves, their families, and other community resources. All of these factors, and others, contribute to and combine with a custodial type of patient care to produce a regressive dependence upon the hospital rather than facilitate the retention and reactivation of the more self-reliant, health-producing potential of patients.

Manpower shortages are an important factor contributing to the problems of patient care and treatment. Perhaps even more significant than the shortages in *numbers* of staff are the limitations of *training* and *experience* of key staff personnel. The latter condition of many state hospital staffs results in exceedingly serious weaknesses of clinical leadership.

Weakness of clinical leadership is indigenous to many if not most state hospitals—particularly those which are geographically remote from population centers and are therefore isolated professionally. One of the severest shortages in such hospitals is that of talented, well-trained psychiatrists.

Surprisingly little attention has been paid to problems of clinical leadership in state hospitals and what might be done about this problem through training programs. Most of the efforts to improve patient care and treatment have emphasized recruitment policies, social psychiatric approaches, such administrative changes as decentralization with the formation of interdisciplinary unit teams and fuller use of ancillary personnel—the latter often without sufficient attention to the training and supervisory needs of those ancillary personnel, upon whom greater responsibilities for patient care and treatment are thrust. In addition, just as the fuller use of ancillary personnel to relieve manpower shortages and to improve patient care has often not been accompanied by a corresponding increase in the amount of training for these personnel, similarly, the increasing integration of ancillary personnel in interdisciplinary teams has usually not been accompanied by special training in collaborative work with heterogeneous groups.

A few promising "laboratory-type" training methods have been developed to deal with these difficult interpersonal problems of group functioning. In such approaches, the staff members making up a particular working team undergo variable periods of supervised participation in training groups, the purpose of which is to improve their ability to function effectively and collaboratively in their "back home" work groups. As the unit system and fuller use of ancillary personnel become more widespread in large psychiatric hospitals, increasing attention will have to be paid to these troublesome problems of people working together in groups. The formation, development, and functioning of consultant teams such as our own present identical group problems. Teams such as ours are by no means immune to these ubiquitous human difficulties of people attempting to work together. In fact, unless these problems are worked out satisfactorily within the training team, the unresolved conflicts and tensions among the consultants are likely to be reflected in training problems and difficulties within the hospital staff and, ultimately, in clinical disturbances among the patients of the hospital. It is incumbent upon a consultant team, therefore, as well as upon clinical teams within a hospital staff, to observe, study, and discuss their own group-process problems ceaselessly and candidly, attempting to diagnose and deal with their interpersonal conflicts as quickly and completely as possible, both to maintain optimal functioning within the consultant or clinical team, and to prevent a "contagion" of their own group problems to other parts of the hospital staff and to patients.

We come finally to the problem of research in state mental hospitals. Like the training needs of these over-sized, understaffed institutions, research appears to be a low priority item in most state hospitals. Various writers have observed that the relative lack of research in state hospitals is usually explained—in part, justifiably—on the basis of the staff's heavy clinical commitments. Research projects and programs in state hospitals, however, can help to improve professional work and patient care in a number of ways. Aside from the intrinsic value of investigative findings in their own right, research activities promote critical thinking and constant self-examination concerning the value and validity of the methods and concepts being used in a particular hospital. Still another advantage of investigative activities in state hospitals is the stimulating and supportive effect research can have upon staff morale. Discouragement in the staff's work appears to be reduced by a more investigative interest in some of the difficult problems they face.

The problems of state hospital psychiatry are numerous and complexly interrelated. In spite of this almost self-evident fact, many of the writings on state hospital psychiatry stress one or another of the various problems to the exclusion of others, and often recommend a single, oversimplified approach as a "solution." An investigation may focus upon the problems of largeness and isolation of these massive institutions, for example, and then recommend either that such hospitals be abolished altogether—without proposing an alternative plan for these many thousands of patients—or may suggest a single, so-called "solution," such as fuller use of ancillary personnel. As we have stressed here, one of the most serious sets of problems in state mental hospitals, i.e., their training and research needs, have received the least attention and improvements.

In keeping with the multiple, complexly interrelated problems of state hospital psychiatry, the present consultant team approach has attempted to adopt and to follow a complex, multifaceted conception of its tasks, goals, and methods of approach—but at the same time has tried to maintain a streamlined simplicity in its operating procedures. Our consultant team approach has attempted to take into consideration and to improve as many of the fundamental problems of state hospital psychiatry as possible by utilizing as many methods of approach as we could bring to bear upon the problems—at the same time recognizing that no matter how comprehensive we might attempt to be, our efforts could never be complete or definitive, but only catalytic in their effects. Finally, in our attempts to do remedial justice rather than reductionistic violence to the complexities of state hospital problems, our consultant team approach has attempted to give high priority to the much neglected but vitally important training and research needs of these institutions, their staffs, and their patients.

Bibliography*

Abea, J. M., & Albright, J. V. (1960), The team approach to psychiatric treatment in a dynamic milieu. *Ment. Hosp.*, 11:30-31 (II A 2; II B 1).

Abroms, G. M. (1969), Defining milieu therapy. *Arch. Gen. Psychiat.*, 21:553-560 (II B 1).

Ackerman, N.W. (1963), Family diagnosis and therapy. In: Masserman, J. H. (Ed.), *Current Psychiatric Therapies*, 3:205-218. N.Y.: Grune & Stratton (II B 4).

Ackerman, O. R., Mitsos, S. B., Seymour, A. M., & Smith, B. K. (1959), Patients go camping in Indiana and in Texas. *Ment. Hosp.*, 10(6):16-18 (II B 2).

Adams, H. B. (1961), The influence of social variables, treatment methods, and administrative factors on mental hospital admission rates. *Psychiat. Quart.*, 35:353-372 (I A 1; I B 2; I C 3; I B 1).

Adland, M. L. (1955), Personnel—effect on patients. *Neuropsychiat.*, 3:110-131 (II A 3 a; I C 3; II B 1; I B 1).

Adorno, T. W., Frenkel-Brunswick, E., Levinson, D. J., & Sanford, R. N. (1950), *The Authoritarian Personality*. N.Y.: Harper (I B 2).

Albee, G. W., & Dickey, M. (1957), Manpower trends in three mental health professions. *Amer. Psychologist*, 12:57-70 (I C 1; I A 2; I A 1; II A 3 a).

Allen, A. (1975), The psychoanalyst and the state hospital. *Dis. Nerv. Syst.* 36:666-669 (II A 3 b).

Allport, D. B. (1943), Religion and state hospital. *Ment. Hygiene*, 27:574 ((II A 3 k).

Almond, R., Keniston, K., & Boltox, R. (1968), The value system of a milieu therapy unit. *Arch. Gen. Psychiat.*, 19:545-561 (II B 1).
—————————————— (1969), Patient value change in milieu therapy. *Arch. Gen. Psychiat.*, 20:339-351 (II B 1).

---

*The numerals, letters, and numbers in parentheses refer to Subject Index categories (see Subject Index, pp. 237-253).

Amenn, L., Berman, S., & Brody, E. B. (1954), *Patient Government*. Information Bulletin 10-70. Wash., D.C.: Dept. Med. & Surg., Veterans Adm. (II B 3).

American Hospital Association (1945-1975), *Hospital Literature Index*. Chicago: Amer. Hosp. Assoc. (See esp. "Psychiatric Hospitals." Published quarterly, each fourth issue being an annual cumulation. Each fifth year the Index is cumulated as, *Cumulative Index of Hospital Literature*. Chicago: Amer. Hosp. Assoc.) (I ABC; II ABC).

American Medical Association (1964), *Community Mental Health Services and Resources*. Proceedings of the second National Congress on Mental Illness and Health, Chicago, Nov. 5-7 (II B 6).

American Psychiatric Association (1950a), *Mental Hospitals*. Proceedings of the second Mental Hospital Institute. Wash., D.C.: Amer. Psychiat. Assoc., Ment. Hosp. Serv. (I A 1).

_____ (1950b), *Psychiatric Nursing Personnel*. Wash., D.C.: Amer. Psychiat. Assoc., Ment. Hosp. Serv. (II A 3 g).

_____ (1951a), *Working Programs in Mental Hospitals*. Proceedings of the third Mental Hospital Institute. Wash., D.C.: Amer. Psychiat. Assoc., Ment. Hosp. Serv. (I A 1; I C 3).

_____ (1951b), *Standards for Psychiatric Hospitals and Clinics*. Wash., D.C.: Amer. Psychiat. Assoc., Ment. Hosp. Serv. Suppl. No. 1, July 1952, rev. 1954 (I A 1).

_____ (1952), *Steps Forward in Mental Hospitals*. Proceedings of the fourth Mental Hospital Institute. Wash., D.C.: Amer. Psychiat. Assoc., Ment. Hosp. Serv. (I A 1; I C 3).

_____ (1959), *The Volunteer and the Psychiatric Patient*. Wash., D.C.: Amer. Psychiat. Assoc. (II A 3 j).

_____ (1960), *Report on Remotivation*. Wash., D.C.: Amer. Psychiat. Assoc., Ment. Hosp. Serv. (I C 3; II A 3 a).

_____ (1962), *A Position Statement with Interpretative Commentary and Commendation Concerning "Action for Mental Health," The Final Report of the Joint Commission on Mental Illness and Health*. Adopted by the Council of the American Psychiatric Association, Jan. 15. Wash., D.C.: Amer. Psychiat. Assoc. (I A 1).

_____ (1963), Opinions of selected mental health authorities regarding the usefulness of a National Service Corps. *Psychiatric Studies and Projects*, No. 2. Wash., D.C.: Amer. Psychiat. Assoc. (II A 3 a).

_____ (1964a), The development of standards and training curriculum for volunteer services coordinators. *Psychiatric Studies and Projects 2,* No. 2. Wash., D.C.: Amer. Psychiat. Assoc. (II C 1; II A 3 j).

―――― (1964b), Emerging patterns of administration in psychiatric facilities. *Psychiatric Studies and Projects 2,* No. 9. Wash., D.C.: Amer. Psychiat. Assoc. (I B 2).

―――― (1968), *Psychiatric Utilization Review: Principles and Objectives.* Wash., D.C.: Amer. Psychiat. Assoc. (I C 3).

―――― (1969), *Standards for Psychiatric Facilities.* Wash., D.C.: Amer. Psychiat. Assoc., rev. 1974 (I A 1).

―――― (1971), *Eleven Indices: An Aid in Reviewing State and Local Mental Health and Hospital Programs.* Wash., D.C.: Amer. Psychiat. Assoc. (I A 1).

American Psychiatric Association & American Hospital Association (joint statement) (1974), Position statement on the need to maintain long-term mental hospital facilities. *Amer. J. Psychiat.,* 131:745 (I A 1).

American Psychiatric Association Task Force (1971), Research aspects of community mental health centers: Report of the APA task force. *Amer. J. Psychiat.,* 127:993-998. (II B 7; II C 2).

American Red Cross (1956), *Service by Red Cross Volunteers in Civilian Mental Hospitals.* N. Y.: American Red Cross (II A 3 j).

Anonymous (1936), Portrait of a hospital. 2. Herrison Hospital, Dorchester. *Nurs. Times,* 59:170-174 (I A 1).

Anonymous (1937), Selected references on social psychiatry. *Amer. J. Sociol.,* 42:892-894 (I B 1; II B 1).

Appleby, L. (1959), Intrusion. (Major weaknesses in mental hospital structure; proposal of alternate method based on social psychological theory.) *J. Kansas Med. Soc.,* 60:173-177 (I B 1).

―――― , Ellis, N. C., Rogers, G. W., & Zimmerman, W. A. (1961), A psychological contribution to the study of a hospital social structure. *J. Clin. Psychol.,* 17:390-393 (I B 1).

Argyris, C. (1962), *Interpersonal Competence and Organizational Effectiveness.* Homewood, Ill.: Irwin-Dorsey (I B 3; II C 1; I B 2; I B 1; I C 2).

Arthur, R. J. (1971), *An Introduction to Social Psychiatry.* London: Penguin Books (II B 1-7).

―――― (1973), Social psychiatry: An overview. *Amer. J. Psychiat.,* 130:841-849 (II B 1-7).

Artiss, K. L., & Schiff, S. B. (1969), Education for practice in the therapeutic community. *Curr. Psychiat. Ther.*, 8:233-247 (II B 1; II C 1).

Allyon, T., & Michael, J. (1959), The psychiatric nurse as a behavioral engineer. *J. Exp. Anal. Behav.*, 2:323-334 (II A 3 g).

Backner, B. L., & Kissinger, R. D. (1963), Hospital patients' attitudes toward mental health professionals and mental patients. *J. Nerv. Ment. Dis.*, 136:72-75 (II B 3; I B 1).

Baer, W. H. (1952), The training of attendants, psychiatric aides and psychiatric technicians. *Amer. J. Psychiat.*, 109:291 (II C 1; II A 3 i).

Baganz, C. N. (1951), Psychiatric aspects of hospital administration. *Amer. J. Psychiat.*, 108:277 (I B 2).

——— (1953), The growing science of mental hospital administration. *Amer. J. Psychiat.*, 110:161 (I B 2).

Baker, A. A. (1963), A medium-stay hospital. *Lancet,* 1:879-890 (I A 1).

——— & Thorpe, J. G. (1956), Deteriorated psychotic patients—their treatment and its assessment. *J. Ment. Sci.*, 102:780-789 (I C 3).

Baker, E. F. (1960), The mental hospital patient in Canada. *Canad. Med. Assoc. J.*, 82:733 (I A 1).

Baker, F. (1966), An open-systems approach to the study of mental hospitals in transition. Presented to the Annual Meeting of the American Psychological Association, N.Y., Sept. 2-6 (II C 2).

——— & Schulberg, H. C. (1967), The development of a community mental health ideology scale. *Commun. Ment. Health J.,* 3:216-225 (II B 7).

Baldwin, J. A. (1963), A critique of the use of patient-movement studies in the planning of mental health services. *Scot. Med. J.,* 8:227-233 (I B 3; II B 1).

Band, R. I., & Brody, E. B. (1962), Human elements in the therapeutic community. *Arch. Gen. Psychiat.*, 6:307-314 (I B 1).

Bandler, B. (1968), The American Psychoanalytic Association and community psychiatry. *Amer. J. Psychiat.*, 124:1037-1042 (II A 3 b; II B 7).

Banks, E. P. (1956), Methodological problems in the study of psychiatric wards. *Soc. Forces,* 34:277-280 (II B 1).

Barchilon, J. (1964), Some conscious and unconscious factors in teaching psychotherapy by watching through one-way screen, TV or movie films. Presented to the Annual Meeting of the American Psychiatric Association, Los Angeles, May 5 (II C 1).

Barker, D., Brown, L. B., Cawte, J. E., & Riley, J. (1958), Revising the patient's stay in a mental hospital. *Med. J. Austral.*, 45:700-702 (I B 1).

Barrabee, P. S. (1951), A study of a mental hospital; the effect of its social structure on its functions. Cambridge, Mass.: Unpublished Ph.D. dissertation, Harvard Univ. (I B 1).

Bartemeier, L. H. (1952), Professional barriers inhibit teamwork. *Ment. Hosp.*, 3:3 (I B 3).

Bartlett, L. L., & Aurnhammer, M. D. (1957), Psychiatric lecture series for all employees. *Ment. Hosp.*, 8:14 (II C 1; II A 3).

Barton, W. E. (1950), The nurse as an active member of the psychiatric team. *Amer. J. Nurs.*, 50:714 (II A 3 g).

———— (1956), A psychiatric team in action. *Ment. Hosp.* 7:3-9 (II A 2).

———— (1962a), The hospital administrator. *Ment. Hosp.*, 13:259-264 (I B 2).

———— (1962b), The future of the mental hospital. The portent of some current emphases. *Ment. Hosp.*, 13:368-369 (I A 1).

———— (1962c), Social therapy and aftercare. In: *World Congress of Psychiatry, Proceedings of the Third Congress*. Toronto: Univ. Toronto Press, pp. 379-380 (II B 1; II B 5).

———— (1963), Mental hospitals in Japan. *Ment. Hosp.*, 14:489-491 (I A 1).

————, Tybring, G. B., Ewalds, R. M., & Gralnick, A. (1962), The future of the mental hospital. *Ment. Hosp.*, 13:2-8 (I A 1).

Bass, R. D., & Windle, C. (1972), Continuity of care: An approach to measurement. *Amer. J. Psychiat.*, 129:196-201 (II B 5; II B 7).

Bateman, J. F., & Dunham, H. W. (1948), The state mental hospital as a specialized community experience. *Amer. J. Psychiat.*, 105: 445-448 (II B 1; I B 1).

Batey, M. V., & Julian, J. (1963), Staff perceptions of state psychiatric hospital goals. *Nurs. Res.*, 12:80-92 (I A 2; I B 1).

Baur, A. K. (1957), Management and a state hospital. *Ment. Hosp.*, 8:8-9 (I B 2).

Bavelas, A. (1948), Some problems of organizational change. *J. Soc. Issues*, 4:48-52 (I B 3; I B 1; I B 2).

Beckenstein, N. (1964), The new state hospital. In: Bellak, L. (Ed.) (1964), pp. 177-188 (II B 6).

Becker, R. E. (1967), An evaluation of a rehabilitation program for chronically hospitalized psychiatric patients. *Soc. Psychiat.*, 2:32-38 (I C 3; II C 2).

———— (1971), Group preparation for discharge and group placement of chronically hospitalized schizophrenic patients. *Dis. Nerv. Syst.*, 32:176-179 (II B 1).

_____ (1975), The effects of clinical treatment conditions on predictors of length of hospital stay. *Dis. Nerv. Syst.*, 36:309-315 (I C 3; II C 2).

Beisser, A. R., Abe, G. Y., & Wyers, R. E. (1959), How residency training affects a state hospital. *Ment. Hosp.*, 10:7-9 (II C 1).

Belknap, I. (1956), *Human Problems of a State Mental Hospital.* N.Y.: McGraw-Hill (I B 1; I A 1; I B 2).

Bell, G. M. (1955), A mental hospital with open doors. *Internat. J. Soc. Psychiat.*, 1:42-48 (II B 2).

Bellak, L. (Ed.) (1964), *Handbook of Community Psychiatry and Community Mental Health.* N. Y.: Grune & Stratton (II B 6).

_____ , Beavers, A., Lehine, D., & Schusdek, A. (1963), Psychiatric training program for nonpsychiatric physicians. *JAMA*, 184:470-472 (II C 1).

Benady, D. R., & Denham, J. (1963), Development of an early treatment unit from an observation ward. *Brit. Med. J.* (Dec. 21): 1569-1572 (I C 3).

Berke, M. (1959), How to staff the psychiatric unit. *Mod. Hosp.*, 93:87-90 (II A 2; II A 1).

Berlin, I. N. (1969), Resistance to change in mental health professionals. *Amer. J. Orthopsychiat.*, 39:110-115 (II B 7).

Berry, E. (1963), A volunteer program penetrates a maximum security setting. *Ment. Hosp.*, 14:503 (II A 3 j).

Bickford, J. A. (1963), Economic value of the psychiatric inpatient. *Lancet*, 1:714-715 (I A 1).

Bierer, J., & Evans, R. I. (1959), *Innovations in Social Psychiatry.* London: Avenue (II B 5).

_____ & Haldane, F. P. (1941), A self-governed patients' social club in a public mental hospital. *J. Ment. Sci.*, 87:419-424 (II B 3).

Bindman, A. J., & Spiegel, A. D. (Eds.) (1970), *Perspectives in Community Mental Health.* Chicago: Aldine (II B 7).

Birnbaum, M. (1975), Recent Supreme Court developments and the goals of the right to treatment. Presented to the Annual Meeting of the American Psychiatric Association, Anaheim, Calif., May 5-9. *Scientific Proceedings in Summary Form.* Wash., D.C.: Amer. Psychiat. Assoc., pp. 173-174 (I C 3).

Bishop, D. C., & Zubowicz, G. (1963), Communication channels for employees. *Ment. Hosp.*, 14:277 (I B 3).

Black, B. J. (1957), The workaday world; some problems in return of mental patients to the community. In: Greenblatt, M.,

Levinson, D. J., & Williams, R. H. (Eds.) (1957), pp. 572-581 (II B 2; II B 6).

Black, K. (1953), *Psychiatric Nursing Today.* Proceedings of the First Annual Psychiatric Institute, N. J. Neuropsychiatric Institute (II A 3 g).

Blain, D. (Ed.) (1949), *Better Care in Mental Hospitals.* Proceedings of the First Annual Institute of the American Psychiatric Association. Wash., D.C.: Amer. Psychiat. Assoc. (I C 3; I A 1).

_____ (1963), Mental health and hospital care in California. *Calif. Med.,* 99:70-73 (I A 1; I C 3).

_____ , Babcock, K. B., & Gerty, F. C. (1963), Psychiatric hospital accreditation. *Ment. Hosp.* 14:115-119 (I A 1).

Blake, R. R., & Mouton, J. S. (1962), The instrumented training laboratory. In: Schein, E., & Weschier, I. (Eds.), *New Trends in Human Relations Training.* Wash., D.C.: Nat. Training Labs.-Nat. Educ. Assoc. (I B 3).

_____ _____ (1963), The induction of change in organizations. Unpublished report, Univ. of Texas (I B 3; I B 2; I B 1).

Blank, H. R. (1960), The multidisciplinary treatment and research team. *New Outlook for the Blind,* 54:115-119 (II A 2).

_____ (1964), Community psychiatry and the psychiatrist in private practice. In: Bellak, L. (Ed.) (1964), pp. 300-318 (II C 3; I C 1; II B 6).

Blasko, J. J. (1962), V.A. hospital units. *Hosp. Progr.,* 43:77-79 (II A 1).

Bloomberg, W. (1960), A proposal for a community-based hospital as a branch of a state hospital. *Amer. J. Psychiat.,* 116:814-817 (II B 6).

_____ & Rockmore, M. J. (1967), The interstate compact on mental health. *Amer. J. Psychiat.,* 124:520-526 (I A 1; I A 2).

Bolman, W. M. (1968), Preventive psychiatry for the family: Theory, approaches, and programs. *Amer. J. Psychiat.,* 125:458-472 (II B 7).

_____ (1972), Community control of the community mental health center: I. Introduction. II. Case examples. *Amer. J. Psychiat.,* 129:173-186 (II B 7).

_____ & Westman, J. C. (1967), Prevention of mental disorder: An overview of current programs. *Amer. J. Psychiat.,* 123:1058-1068 (II B 7).

Bond, E. D. (1947), *Dr. Kirkbride and His Mental Hospital.* Philadelphia: Lippincott (I A 1).

———— (1956), Therapeutic forces in early American hospitals. *Amer. J. Psychiat.*, 113:407-408 (I C 3; I A 1).

Bonn, E. M. (1969), A therapeutic community in an open state hospital — administrative-therapeutic links. *Hosp. & Commun. Psychiat.*, 20:269-278 (II B 1; II B 2).

Bonner, C. A., & Taylor, L. E. (1939), A study of accidents in a mental hospital. *Amer. J. Psychiat.*, 96:283 (I A 1).

Bonner, L. A. (1949), Mental hospital employees, their importance in future mental hospital betterment. *Amer. J. Psychiat.*, 105: 669-672 (II A 3).

Boquet, R. F. (1964), Community placement ward: A total team effort. *Ment. Hosp.* 15:320-330 (II B 5; II B 6; II A 2).

Borsch, R. N. (1963), Coping with reassignment anxiety. *Ment. Hosp.* 14:312-316 (II C 1; I B 3).

Bosworth, J. C. (1959), Developing a procedures manual. *Ment. Hosp.* 10(5):38-39 (I B 2; II C 1).

Botts, H. H. (1959), A public relations program for mental hospitals. *Hosp. Manag.*, 35:42-43 (II B 6; I B 1).

Boudwin, J. W., & Garlington, W. K. (1959), An admission ward as a therapeutic community. *Northwest Med.*, 58:223-226 (II B 1).

Bourke, W. W. (1964), Unit system in VA psychiatric hospitals. Presented to the Annual Meeting of the American Psychiatric Association, Los Angeles, May 8 (II A 1).

Bovard, E. W. (1951), The psychology of classroom interaction. *J. Educ. Res.*, 45:215-224 (II C 1; I B 3).

Bowen, M. (1961), The family as the unit of study and treatment. *Amer. J. Orthopsychiat.*, 31:40-60 (II B 4).

Boyd, R. W., Baker, T., & Greenblatt, M. (1954), Ward social behavior: An analysis of patient interaction at highest, lowest extreme. *Nurs. Res.*, 3:77-79 (II B 3; I B 1).

Braceland, F. J. (1956), The future of the mental hospital. *J. Amer. Hosp. Assoc.*, 30:42-45 (I A 1).

———— (1962), A scientific and professional framework for hospital psychiatry. *Hosp. Progr.*, 43:76-81 (I A 2; II C 1).

Bradford, L. P. (1953), *Explorations in Human Relations Training, National Training Laboratory in Group Development, 1947-1953*. Wash., D.C.: Nat. Training Labs.-Nat. Educ. Assoc. (I B 3; II C 1).

———— (Ed.)(1961), *Group Development*. Wash., D.C.: Nat. Training Labs.-Nat. Educ. Assoc. (I B 3; II C 1).

———— (1963), Theory and method in laboratory training. In: Bradford, L. P., Gibb, J. R., & Benne, K. D. (Eds.) (1963) (I B 3; II C 1).

———, Gibb, J. R., & Benne, K. D. (Eds.) (1963), *T-Group Theory and Laboratory Method.* N.Y.: Wiley (I B 3; II C 1).

Bradshaw, F. J., Jr. (1962), Member-employee program as a means of rehabilitation. *Ment. Hygiene,* 46:573-579 (II B 3).

Braginsky, B. M., Braginsky, D. D., & Ring, K. (1969), *Methods of Madness: The Mental Hospital as a Last Resort.* N.Y.: Holt, Rinehart & Winston (I A 1).

Branch, C. H. (1963a), Legal problems related to the care of the mentally ill. The backlash of a broken chain. *New. Engl. J. Med.,* 269:137-142 (II B 2).

——— (1963b), How broad can a hospital program be? *Ment. Hosp.* 14:56-60 (I C 3; II B 6; II B 5).

Branchi, J. T., Eaton, M. T., Jr., & Greaves, D. C. (1961), Future of psychiatry. The theory of the open ward. *J. Kansas Med. Soc.,* 62:107-108 (II B 2).

Bravos, T. A. (1959), Administrative residencies. *Ment. Hosp.,* 10(5): 37 (II C 1; I B 2).

Breggin, P. R. (1964), Coercion of voluntary patients in an open hospital. *Arch. Gen. Psychiat.,* 10:173-181 (II B 2; I C 3).

Brickman, H. R. (1967a), Community mental health—means or end? *Psychiat. Digest,* 28:43-50 (II B 7).

——— (1967b), Community mental health—the metropolitan view. *Amer. J. Public Health,* 57:641-650 (II B 7).

——— (1968), The new mental health system. *Calif. Med.,* 109: 403-408 (II B 7).

——— (1970), Mental health and social change: An ecological perspective. *Amer. J. Psychiat.,* 127:413-419 (II B 7).

———, Schwartz, D. A., & Doran, S. M. (1966), The psychoanalyst as community psychiatrist. *Amer. J. Psychiat.,* 122:1081-1087 (II A 3 b; II B 7).

Briggs, D. L., & Wood, N. R. (1956), Advances in training neuropsychiatric technicians. *U.S. Armed Forces Med. J.,* 7:1615-1620 (II C 1; II A 2).

Brill, H. (1975a), The future of the mental hospital and its patients. *Psychiat. Ann.,* 5:9-21 (I A 1).

——— (1975b), Institutional psychiatry. In: Arieti, S. (Ed.), *New Dimensions in Psychiatry: A World View.* N.Y.: Wiley (I A 1).

———, Folsom, J. C., St. Pierre, R. G., & Zubowicz, G. (1963), The unit system of operation. *Ment. Hosp.,* 14:117-118 (II A 1).

——— & Patton, R. E. (1962), Clinical-statistical analysis of population changes in New York mental hospitals since introduction of psychotropic drugs. *Amer. J. Psychiat.,* 119:20-35 (I A 1; I C 3).

——— ——— (1964), The impact of modern chemotherapy on hospital organization, psychiatric care and public health policies: Its scope and its limits. *Proceedings of Third World Conference on Psychiatry,* Vol. III. Toronto: Univ. Toronto Press, pp. 433-437 (I A 1).

Brockbank, R. (1971), The contributions of psychoanalytical theory to community mental health. *Brit. J. Med. Psychol.,* 44:319-328 (II B 7; II A 3 b).

Brodey, W. (1955), Some family operations and schizophrenia. *Arch. Gen. Psychiat.,* 1:379-402 (II B 4).

Brody, D. S., Sexsmith, H. S., & Sexsmith, D. G. (1960), Teacher education in a mental hospital. *Ment. Hosp.,* 11:48-49 (II C 1).

Brody, E. B. (1960), The public mental hospital as a symptom of social conflict. *Maryland Med. J.,* 9:330 (I B 1; II B 6).

———— (1964), Some conceptual and methodological issues involved in research on society, culture and mental illness. *J. Nerv. Ment. Dis.,* 139: 62-64 (II C 2).

Bromet, E. J. (1971), The post-hospital adjustment of psychiatric patients. New Haven: Unpublished doctoral dissertation, Dept. Public Health & Epidemiol., Yale Univ. (II B 5).

Brooke, E. M. (1962), Factors affecting the demand for psychiatric beds. *Lancet,* 2:1211-1213 (I A 1).

———— (1963), A cohort study of patients first admitted to mental hospitals in 1954 and 1955. London: H. M. Stationery Office (I A 1).

Brooks, G. W. (1961), Effective use of ancillary personnel in rehabilitating the mentally ill. *Texas J. Med.,* 57:341-347 (II A 3).

———— , Deane, W. N., Lagor, R. C., & Curtis, B. B. (1963), Varieties of family participation in the rehabilitation of released chronic schizophrenic patients. *J. Nerv. Ment. Dis.,* 136:432-444 (II B 4).

Brown, B. S. (1963), Pathways and detours to and from the mental hospital. *Missouri Med.,* 60:253-256 (II B 6).

Brown, E. L. (1957), Staff accord must be reached to attain hospital objectives. *Ment. Hosp.,* 8:16-19 (I B 3).

———— , Dunham, H. W., & York, R. H. (1957), The application of the sciences of social behavior in ward settings. In: Greenblatt, M., Levinson, D. J., & Williams, R. H. (Eds.) (1957), pp. 479-498 (I B 1).

Brown, G. W. (1960), Length of hospital stay and schizophrenia: Review of statistical studies. *Acta. Psychiat. Scand.,* 35:414-430 (I A 1; I C 3).

———— , Parkes, C. M., & Wing, J. K. (1961), Admissions and re-admissions to three London mental hospitals. *J. Ment. Sci.*, 107: 1070-1077 (I A 1).

Bruder, E. E. (1953), A ministry to the mentally ill in the mental hospital. In: Maves, P. B. (Ed.), *The Church and Mental Health.* N.Y.: Scribner (II A 3 k).

Brunt, H. H. (1959), Patients promote community relations. *Ment. Hosp.*, 10:16 (II B 3; II B 6).

Bryan, W. (1936), *Administrative Psychiatry.* N.Y.: Norton (I B 2).

Bullard, D. M. (1952), Problems of clinical administration. *Bull. Menninger Clin.*, 16:193-201 (I B 2).

Bunker, H. A. (1944), American psychiatric literature during the past one hundred years. In: *American Psychiatry, 1844-1944.* N.Y.: Columbia Univ. Press (I A 1; I C 3).

Burdock, E. I., Glass, L., Hardesty, A. S., & Beck, Y. M. (1961), A sample survey of mental hospital patients. *J. Clin. Psychol.*, 17: 253-259 (I A 1).

Bureau of the Census (1941), *Patients in Mental Institutions.* Wash., D.C.: Dept. of Commerce (I A 1).

Burrows, W. G. (1969), Community psychiatry—another band-wagon? *Canad. Psychiat. Assoc. J.*, 14:105-114 (II B 7).

Bush, C. K. (1959a), How the Central Inspection Board rates facilities for patient care. *Ment. Hosp.*, 10(5):22-23 (I C 3; I A 1).

———— (1959b), Why organize the medical staff? *Ment. Hosp.*, 10:26 (I C 2; II A 2).

———— (1960a), Hospital administration. *Ment. Hosp.*, 11:48 (I B 2).

———— (1960b), Nursing service criteria. *Ment. Hosp.*, 11:13 (II A 3 g).

Butkiewicz, R. M., & Fields, J. F. (1960), A teaching device for nursing students. *Ment. Hosp.*, 11:47 (II C 1; II A 3 g).

Butler, H. S., & Flood, F. R. (1962), Evaluating nursing care in a mental hospital. *Amer. J. Nurs.*, 62:84-85 (II A 3 g).

Cameron, D. E. (1950), Modern methods of treatment require an open psychiatric hospital. *Mod. Hosp.*, 74:84-88 (II B 2).

———— (1951), The day hospital: An approach to expanding hospital facilities. In: *Mental Hospitals, 1950: Proceedings of the Second Mental Hospital Institute.* Wash., D.C.: Amer. Psychiat. Assoc. (II B 5).

———— (1963), Treatment in public mental hospitals. *Ment. Hosp.*, 14:80-87 (I C 3).

Cameron, J. L. (1963), Patient, therapist and administrator: Clinical and theoretical investigation of a conflictual situation. *Brit. J. Med. Psychol.*, 36:13-25 (I B 3; I B 2; I C 3).

Canadian Mental Health Association (1962), *High Road to Mental Health—Summary, Highlights and Recommendations of the Five-Year Study of Psychiatric Treatment Services in Canada.* Toronto: Canad. Ment. Health Assoc. (I C 3; I A 1).

Cancro, R. (1969), Prospective prediction of hospital stay in schizophrenia. *Arch. Gen. Psychiat.*, 20:541-546 (II C 2).

_____ (1970), A review of current research directions: Their product and their promise. The schizophrenic reactions: A critique of the concept, hospital treatment and current research. N.Y.: Brunner/Mazel, pp. 189-196 (II C 2).

Caplan, G. (1961), *An Approach to Community Mental Health.* N.Y.: Grune & Stratton (II B 7).

_____ (1967), *Principles of Preventive Psychiatry.* N.Y.: Basic Books (II B 7).

Capoore, H. S., Lieberman, D. M., Norton, A. R., & Tewfik, G. I. (1960), A plan for medical administration in mental hospitals. *Brit. Med. J. Suppl.*, 2881:195-196. In: *Brit. Med. J.*, 5179 (I B 2).

Carson, R. C., Margolis, P. M., Daniels, R. S., & Heine, R. W. (1962), Milieu homogeneity in the treatment of psychiatric inpatients. *Psychiatry,* 25:285-289 (II B 1; I C 3).

Carstairs, G. M., & Heron, A. (1957), The social environment of mental hospital patients: A measure of staff attitudes. In: Greenblatt, M., Levinson, D. J., & Williams, R. H. (Eds.) (1957), pp. 218-230 (I B 1; II B 1).

Carter, F. M. (1959), The critical incident technique in identification of the patients' perception of therapeutic patient-patient interaction on a psychiatric hospital ward. *Nurs. Res.*, 8:207-211 (II B 3; II C 2).

Cartwright, D. (Ed.) (1959), *Studies in Social Power.* Ann Arbor: Research Center for Group Dynamics, Inst. Soc. Research, Univ. of Mich. (I B 2; I B 1; I C 2).

_____ & Zander, A. (1953), The structural properties of groups. In: Cartwright, D., & Zander, A. (Eds.), *Group Dynamics.* Evanston: Row, Peterson (I B 3; I B 1).

Carty, R. C., & Breault, G. C. (1967), Gheel: A comprehensive community mental health program. *Perspect. Psychiat. Care,* 5:281-285 (II B 1; II B 7).

Caudill, W. (1956), Perspectives on administration in psychiatric hospitals. *Admin. Sci. Quart.*, 1:155-170 (I B 2; I B 1).

_____ (1957), Social processes in a collective disturbance on a psychiatric ward. In: Greenblatt, M., Levinson, D. J., & Williams, R. H. (Eds.) (1957), pp. 438-471 (I B 1).

—— (1958), *The Psychiatric Hospital as a Small Society.* Cambridge, Mass.: Harvard Univ. Press (I B 1).

——, Redlich, F. C., Gilmore, H. R., & Brody, E. B. (1952), Social structure and interaction processes on a psychiatric ward. *Amer. J. Orthopsychiat.,* 22:314-334 (I B 1).

—— & Stainbrook, E. (1954), Some covert effects of communication difficulties in a psychiatric hospital. *Psychiatry,* 17:27-40 (I B 1; I B 3).

Cawte, J. E., & Brown, L. B. (1962), Assent and dissent in an unlocked mental hospital. *Med. J. Austral.,* 49:644-646 (II B 2).

Chasin, R. M. (1967), Special clinical problems in day hospitalization. *Amer. J. Psychiat.,* 123:779-785 (II B 5).

Chessick, R. D., Wasserman, E. M., Huels, M., & Gerty, F. J. (1959), The psychiatric ward administrator. *Ment. Hosp.* 10(3):7-10 (I C 2).

Christie, P. (1962), Administration and therapy. A survey of processes. *Canad. Psychiat. Assoc. J.,* 7:34-43 (I B 2).

Christie, R., & Jahoda, M. (Eds.) (1954), Authoritarianism reexamined. In: *Studies in the Scope and Method of "The Authoritarian Personality."* Glencoe, Ill.: Free Press (I B 2).

Christmas, J. J., & Davis, E. B. (1965), Group therapy programs with the socially deprived in community psychiatry. *Internat. J. Group Psychother.,* 15:464-476 (II B 1; II B 7).

Chu, F. D., & Trotter, S. (1974), *The Madness Establishment.* N.Y.: Grossman (I A 1).

Clancey, I. L. (1959), Therapeutic aspects of the mental hospital organization. *Canad. Psychiat. Assoc. J.,* 11:7-8 (I B 1; II B 1).

—— (1960), Primary functions in a mental hospital. *Ment. Hosp.,* 11:20-25 (I C 3).

—— & Osmond, H. (1959), Permissive and authoritarian: Two misleading words. *Ment. Hosp.* 10(4):35 (I B 3).

Clark, D. H. (1960), Principles of administrative therapy. *Amer. J Psychiat.,* 117:506-510 (I B 2; II B 1).

—— (1962), Mental hospitals open their doors. *Lancet* 82:145-149 (II B 2).

—— (1963), Administrative psychiatry, 1942-1962. *Brit. J. Psychiat.,* 109:178-201 (I B 2).

Clausen, J. A., & Radke, M. (1955), Paths to the mental hospital. *J. Soc. Issues,* 11:25-32 (II B 6).

Clayton, T. (1974), The changing mental hospital: Emerging alternatives. *Hosp. & Commun. Psychiat.,* 25:386-392.

Cleland, C. C., & Chambers, W. R. (1959), Experimental modification of attitudes as a function of an institutional tour. *Amer. J. Ment. Def.,* 64:124-130 (I B 1).

Coch, L., & French, J. R. P., (1948), Overcoming resistance to change. *Human Relations,* 1:512-532 (I B 1; I B 2).

Cohen, C. I., Sichel, W., & Berger, D. (1975), Breaking the revolving door syndrome. Presented to the Annual Meeting of the American Psychiatric Association, Anaheim, Calif., May 5-9. *Scientific Proceedings in Summary Form.* Wash., D.C.: Amer. Psychiat. Assoc., pp. 217-218 (II B 6).

Cohen, R. A. (1958), The hospital as a therapeutic instrument. *Psychiatry,* 2:29 (I C 3).

Cole, N. J., Brewer, D. L., Allison, R. B., & Branch, C. H. (1964), Employment characteristics of discharged schizophrenics. *Arch. Gen. Psychiat.,* 10:314-319 (II B 5).

Coleman, J. V. (1950), Contribution of the psychiatrist to the clinical team. In: *Education for Psychiatric Social Work.* N.Y.: Amer. Assoc. Psychiat. Soc. Workers (II A 3c; I C 2).

———— (1967), A community project in behalf of the hospitalized mentally ill patient: The cooperative care project. *Amer. J. Psychiat.,* 124:76-79 (II B 6).

———— (1971), Community psychiatry: A change in course. *Amer. J. Psychiat.,* 127:938-939 (II B 7).

Collarelli, N. J., & Siegel, S. M. (1963), Administrative structure and treatment goals: Dysrhythmia? *Ment. Hosp.,* 14 (Nov.) (I B 1).

Colman, A., & Greenblatt, M. (1963), Are beds becoming obsolete? *Amer. J. Nurs.,* 63:60-64 (I A 1).

Cone, W. (1964), The therapeutic community in action: A St. Louis experience. In: Wessen, A. F. (1964), pp. 147-168 (II B 1).

Connery, M. F. (1951), Problems in teaching the team concept. *J. Psychiat. Soc. Work,* 21:81-89 (II A 2; II C 1).

Conran, P. (1962), A practical therapeutic ward milieu. *Dis. Nerv. Syst.,* 23:562-564 (II B 1).

Conte, W. R. (1960), The state psychiatric hospitals and the state medical association: A plan for cooperative efforts. *Northwest Med.,* 59:341-342 (I A 2; II B 6; II A 3 a).

———— & Liebes, R. (1960), *A Voluntary Partnership.* Austin, Tex.: Hogg Found. Mental Health, Univ. of Texas (II A 3 j).

Cook, E. C. (1960), Ward management in a state hospital. *Ment. Hosp.* 11:25-27 (I C 2; I B 2).

Costello, C. G., & Gazan, M. (1962), Desegregation in a psychiatric unit. *Canad. Nurse,* 58:1098-1100 (I C 3; II B 1).

Cote, F., Dancey, T. E., & Saucier, J. (1954), Participation in institutional treatment by selected relatives. *Amer. J. Psychiat.*, 111:831 (II B 4).

Council of Social Work Education (1961), Building the social work curriculum. Report of the National Curriculum Workshop, Allerton, Ill., June 13-18, 1960. N.Y.: Council on Soc. Work Educ. (II C 1; II A 3 f).

Council of State Governments (1950), *The Mental Health Programs of the Forty-Eight States.* Chicago: Council of State Govts. (I A 1).

———— (1953), *Training and Research in State Mental Health Programs.* Chicago: Council of State Govts. (See esp. Chap. 1 for general problems of mental hospitals.) (II C 1; II C 2; I A 1).

Cowen, J. R., & Schwartz, L. (1960), An experiment in the utilization of a clinical psychologist as a ward clinical administrator in a state psychiatric hospital. *Psychiat. Quart.*, 34:472-479 (I C 2; II A 3 e).

Craft, M. (1959), Psychiatric day hospitals. *Amer. J. Psychiat.*, 116:251-253 (II B 5).

Crawshaw, R. (1958), Team operation study. In: *A Study in Adjunctive Therapies Coordination.* Topeka: Washburn Univ. (II A 2; I B 3).

———— & Key, W. (1961), Psychiatric teams—a selective review of the literature. *Arch. Gen. Psychiat.*, 5:397-405 (II A 2).

Croog, S. H. (1956), Patient government: Some aspects of participation and social background on two psychiatric wards. *Psychiatry*, 19:203-207 (II B 3).

Cruvant, B. A. (1953), The function of the "administrative group" in a mental hospital group therapy program. *Amer. J. Psychiat.*, 110:342 (I C 2; I C 3).

Cumming, E. (1962), Phase movement in the support and control of the psychiatric patient. *J. Health. Hum. Behav.*, 3:235-241 (I C 3; II B 1; I B 1).

———— Clancey, I. L. W., & Cumming, J. (1956), Improving patient care through organizational changes in the mental hospital. *Psychiatry*, 19:249-262 (I B 1; I B 2; I C 3).

———— & Cumming, J. (1956), The locus of power in a large mental hospital. *Psychiatry*, 19:261-369 (I B 1; I B 2; I C 2).

———— ———— (1957a), *Closed Ranks.* Cambride, Mass.: Commonwealth Fund. Harvard Univ. Press (I C 1; II B 6).

———— ———— (1957b), Social equilibrium and social change in the large mental hospital. In: Greenblatt, M., Levinson, D. J., & Williams, R. H. (Eds.) (1957), pp. 49-55 (I B 1).

Cumming, J., & Cumming, E. (1962), *Ego and Milieu*. N.Y.: Ather ton (II B 1; I B 1).

Curry, A. E. (1959), Developing a training program for industrial personnel. *Ment. Hosp.*, 10(4):40-41 (II C 1; II A 3 h).

Curtis, C. (1961), Nursing programs in the open hospital. *Ment. Hosp.*, 12:60-61 (II B 2; II A 3 g).

Curtis, W. R. (1973), Community human service networks: New roles for mental health workers. *Psychiat. Ann.*, 3:23-42 (II B 7).

Daniels, R. S. (1962), Education and training within and without the hospital. *Hosp. Progr.*, 42:115-118 (II C 1; II B 6; II C 3).

Darley, P. J., & Kenny, W. T. (1971), Community care and the "Queequeg syndrome": A phenomenological evaluation of methods of rehabilitation for psychotic patients. *Amer. J. Psychiat.*, 127:1333-1338 (II B 7).

Davidson, H. A. (1959), Make your statistics speak English. *Ment. Hosp.*, 10(3):39-40 (I A 1).

_____ & Russell, J. D. (1963), The mental hospital. *Ment. Hosp.*, 14:109-110 (I A 1).

Davies, T. S. (1962), Closed-circuit television in a mental hospital. *Brit. Med. J.*, 5318:1531-1532 (II C 1).

Davis, F. (1960), Uncertainty in medical prognosis, clinical and functional. *Amer. J. Sociol.*, 66:41-47 (I C 2).

Davis, J. A., Freeman, H. E., & Simmons, O.G. (1957), Rehospitalization and performance levels among former mental patients. *Soc. Probs.*, 5:37-44 (I A 1; II B 3).

Davis, J. E. (1957), Research as part of every hospital program. *Ment. Hosp.*, 8:34-36 (II C 2).

_____ & Tolor, A. (1959), Aggressive behavior of staff members in a neuropsychiatric setting. *Ment. Hygiene,* 43:545;554 (I B 1; I B 3).

Deane, W. N. (1961), The reactions of a non-patient to a stay on a mental hospital ward. *Psychiatry,* 24:61-68 (I B 1).

Deasy, L., & Quinn, O. W. (1955), The wife of the mental patient and the hospital psychiatrist. *J. Soc. Issues,* 11:49-60 (II B 4).

Delange, W. H. (1962), Conceptions of patient role by patients and staff in a state mental hospital. *Compr. Psychiat.*, 3:174-180 (I B 1).

Delay, J., Maisonneune, J., & Benda, P. (1958), Psychosociological research on mental patients in an open ward. *Ann. Med. Psychol. Paris,* 116:417-440 (I B 1; II B 2).

Denber, H. C. B. (1960a), A study of the therapeutic community. In: Masserman, J. H., & Moreno, J .R. (Eds.), *Progress in Psychotherapy*, 5:116-121. N.Y.: Grune & Stratton (II B 1).

———— (1960b), A therapeutic community: Analysis of its operation after two years. In: Denber, H. C. B. (Ed.), *Research Conference on Therapeutic Community*. Springfield, Ill.: Charles C Thomas (II B 1).

———— (1963), Group process in a state hospital. *Amer. J. Orthopsychiat.*, 33:990-911 (I B 3; I B 1).

Denton, P. R. (1959), The mobile psychiatric clinic of the Department of Mental Hygiene and Hospitals. *Virginia Med. Monthly*, 86:534-535 (II C 3; II B 6).

Department of Health, Education, and Welfare (1954), *Care of the Long Term Patient*. Wash., D.C.: Dept. HEW (I C 1; I C 3; I A 2).

———— (1960), *Patients in Mental Institutions*. Wash., D.C.: Dept. HEW, part 3, p. 12 (I A 1).

Detre, T., & Tucker, G. J. (1971), Psychotherapy for the mentally ill: A redefinition of goals. In: Abroms, G., & Greenfield, N.S. (Eds.), *The New Hospital Psychiatry*. N.Y.: Academic Press, pp. 57-65 (I C 3).

Deutsch, A. (1949), *The Mentally Ill in America*. N.Y.: Columbia Univ. Press (I A 1).

Devereux, G. (1944), The social structure of a schizophrenic ward and its therapeutic fitness. *J. Clin. Psychopath.*, 6:231-265 (I B 1; I C 3).

———— (1949), The social structure of the hospital as a factor in total therapy. *Amer. J. Orthopsychiat.*, 19:492-500 (I B 1; I C 3).

De Witt, H. B. (1948), The function of the social worker in the total treatment program in a state mental hospital. *Amer. J. Psychiat.*, 105:298-303 (II A 3 f).

Dickson, J. T. (1949), The contribution of social workers to the interviewing skills of psychologists. *J. Soc. Casework*, 30:318-342 (II A 3 f; II A 3 e; II C 1; I B 3).

Dinitz, S., et al. (1961), Psychiatric and social attributes as predictors of case outcome in mental hospitalization. *Soc. Probs.*, 8:383 (II C 2).

————, Lefton, M., Simpson, J. E., Pasamanick, B., & Patterson, R. M. (1958a), The ward behavior of psychiatrically ill patients. In: *Psychiatric Research Reports*, No. 10. Wash., D.C.: Amer. Psychiat. Assoc., pp. 62-71 (II B 3; II B 1; I B 1).

————, ————, ————, Patterson, R. M., & Pasamanick, B.

(1958b), Correlates and consequences of patient interaction and isolation in a mental hospital. *J. Nerv. Ment. Dis.*, 127:437-442 (II B 3; I B 1; I C 3).

Doban, J. L. (1957), Development of a student volunteer program in a state mental hospital. In: Greenblatt, M., Levinson, D. J., & Williams, R. H. (Eds.) (1957), pp. 593-603 (II A 3 j).

Doehme, E. F., Phillips, R. D., & Sandifer, M. G., Jr. (1964), A study of rehabilitative potential among "chronic" patients in North Carolina mental hospitals. Presented to the Annual Meeting of the American Psychiatric Association, Los Angeles, May 6 (I A 1; I C 3).

Downing, J. (1958), Chronic mental hospital dependency as a character defense. *Psychiat. Quart.*, 32:489-499 (I C 3; I C 1).

Duhl, L. J. (1967), What mental health services are needed for the poor? In: Greenblatt, M., Emory, P. E., & Glueck, B.C. (Eds.), Poverty and mental health. *Psychiat. Res. Rep. Amer. Psychiat. Assoc.*, 21:72-78 (II B 7).

_____ & Leopold, R. L. (Eds.) (1968), *Mental Health and Urban Social Policy*. San Francisco: Jossey-Bass (II B 7).

Dumont, M., Daniels, R. S., Margolis, P. M., Carson, R. C., & Ham, J. (1960), Patient and staff reactions to a change in procedure on a psychiatric ward. *Dis. Nerv. Syst.*, 21:209-212 (I B 1).

Dunham, H. W. (1965), Community psychiatry: The newest therapeutic bandwagon. *Internat. J. Psychiat.*, 1:553-584 (II B 7).

_____ & Meltzer, B. N. (1946), Predicting length of hospitalization of mental patients. *Amer. J. Sociol.*, 52:123-131 (I A 1; I B 1).

_____ & Weinberg, S. K. (1960), *The Culture of the State Mental Hospital*. Detroit: Wayne State Univ. Press (I B 1).

Dunlop, E. (1947), The integration of services in the rehabilitation process. *Occup. Ther. Rehab.*, 26:137 (I C 3; II A 2; I B 3).

Duval, A. M. (1950), The clinical director looks at the hospital superintendent. *Amer. J. Psychiat.* 107:173 (I C 2; I B 2; I B 3).

_____ (1957), Management and the public mental hospital. *Ment. Hosp.*, 8:5-9 (I B 2).

_____ (1963), Dynamic forces in the public mental hospital. *Ment. Hygiene*, 47:3-11 (I B 1).

Dykens, J. W. (1960), The clinical director: Dynamic psychiatrist and scientific manager. *Ment. Hosp.*, 11:50-52 (I C 2; I B 2).

_____ (1963), Recruiting mental hospital workers. *Ment. Hosp.* 14:538-540 (I C 1; I A 2).

_____, Hyde, R. W., Orzack, L. H., & York, R. H. (1964), *Strategies of Mental Hospital Change*. Boston: Commonwealth of

Mass., Dept. of Ment. Health (II C 3; I B 1; I B 2; II C 2).

Eberhart, E. T. (1963), The chaplain as the patients' pastor. *Ment. Hosp.*, 14:271-272 (II A 3).

Edelson, D. (1960), From custodial care to the open psychiatric hospital—a study of the process of effecting administrative and therapeutic change. Evanston, Ill.: Master's thesis in hospital administration, Northwestern Univ. (II B 2; I B 2; I C 3).

Edelson, M. (1964), *Ego Psychology, Group Dynamics, and the Therapeutic Community*. N.Y.: Grune & Stratton (I B 3; II B 1; I C 3).

Editorial comment (1958), Open doors. *Brit. Med. J.*, 5105:1150-1151 (II B 2).

———— (1959a), New concepts of personnel; needs are changing. *Ment. Hosp.*, 10(2):13-15 (II A 3; I C 1).

———— (1959b), Organizing to meet new deeds. *Ment. Hosp.*, 10(2): 15-17 (I B 2).

———— (1959c), Training of ward personnel. *Ment. Hosp.*, 10(2): 18-20 (II C 1; II A 3 i).

———— (1959d), Full utilization of ancillary personnel. *Ment. Hosp.*, 10(2):21-23 (II A 3).

———— (1959e), Recruiting and retaining personnel. *Ment. Hosp.*, 10(2):24-26 (I C 1; I A 2; II C 1).

———— (1959f), Psychoanalytic contributions to treatment programs in mental hospitals. *Ment. Hosp.*, 10(2):50-53 (II A 3 b; I C 3; I A 2; I C 1; II C 1).

———— (1959g), Psychiatry and local authorities. *Lancet*, 1:728 (II B 6).

———— (1963), Psychiatric beds. *Lancet*, 1:369-370 (I A 1).

Edwalds, R. M. (1962), The future of the mental hospital: A dilemma for the young doctor. *Ment. Hosp.*, 13:372-373 (I C 1; I A 2; I C 2).

Eichert, A. N. (1944), Morale and the attendant; a note on the personnel problems in hospitals for the mentally disordered. *Ment. Hygiene*, 28:632-638 (I C 1; II A 3 i; II C 1).

Eichorn, H., & Hyde, R. W. (1950), Friendly and unfriendly interactions in the mental hospital. In: Sorokin, P. A. (Ed.), *Explorations in Altruistic Love and Behavior*. Boston: Beacon Press, Chap. 12 (I B 3; I B 1).

Eiden, V. M. (1963), The modern psychiatric treatment program at Willmar State Hospital. *Lancet*, 83:59-62 (I C 3).

Eisen, A., Lurie, A., & Robbins, L. L. (1963), Group processes in a voluntary psychiatric hospital. *Amer. J. Orthopsychiat.*, 33: 750-754 (I B 3; I B 1; II B 1; II B 2).

Eisenberg, L. (1973), Developments in psychiatric postgraduate training in the United States. *Soc. Sci. Med.*, 7:99-102 (II C 1).

Ekman, P. (1961), Research as therapy. *J. Nerv. Ment. Dis.*, 133· 229-232 (II C 2).

Eliasoph, E. (1959), The use of volunteers as case aides in a treatment setting. *Soc. Casework*, 40:141-144 (II A 3 j; I C 3).

Ellenberger, H. F. (1960), Zoological garden and mental hospital. *Canad. Psychiat. Assoc. J.* 5:136-149 (II B 2).

Ellsworth, R. L., Mead, B. T., & Clayton, W. H. (1958), The rehabilitation and disposition of chronically ill schizophrenic patients. *Ment. Hygiene,* 42:343-348 (I C 3).

Erikson, K. T. (1955), Drama and the role of the patient: Rehearsal for normalcy. Chicago: Unpublished Master's thesis, Univ. of Chicago (I B 1; I C 3).

_____ (1957), Patient role and social uncertainty— a dilemma of the mentally ill. *Psychiatry*, 22:263-274 (I B 1).

Etzioni, A. (1960), Interpersonal and structural factors in the study of mental hospitals. *Psychiatry,* 23:13-22 (I B 1; II C 2).

Ewalt, J. R. (1953), Mental health problems affecting social relations. *Ann. Amer. Polit. Soc. Sci.,* 286:74-80 (I B 3; II B 6).

_____ (1956), *Mental Health Administration*. Springfield, Ill.: Charles C Thomas (I B 2).

_____ , Alexander, G. L., & Grinspoon, L. L. (1960), Changing practices: A plea and some predictions. *Ment. Hosp.,* 11:9-13 (I A 1; I C 3).

Fairweather, G. W., Sanders, D. H., Maynard, H., et al. (1969), *Community Life for the Mentally Ill: An Alternative to Institutional Care*. Chicago: Aldine (II B 7).

Farberow, N. L. (1969), Training in suicide prevention for professional and community agents. *Amer. J. Psychiat.,* 125:1702-1705 (II B 7).

Fechner, A. H., & Parke, J. H. (1951), The volunteer worker and the psychiatric hospital. *Amer. J. Psychiat.,* 107:602 (II A 3 j).

Fein, R. (1958), *Economics of Mental Illness*. N.Y.: Basic Books (I A 1).

Feldman, P. E. (1952), A public health program in a state hospital. *Ment. Health Bull.,* 30:1 (I C 3; I A 1).

Feldman, S. (1971), Ideas and issues in community mental health. *Hosp. & Commun. Psychiat.,* 22:325-329 (II B 7).

Feldstein, E. I. (1939), Psychoanalytic concepts and state hospital psychiatry. *Elgin Papers* 3:105-115 (I C 3; II A 3 b).

Felix, R. H. (1961), The hospital and the community. *Ment. Hosp.*, 12:1-4 (II B 6).

Felzer, S. B., Shumaker, E., D'Zmura, T. L, & Slutsky, H. (1964), A psychiatric training program for community agency personnel. Presented to the Divisional Meeting, American Psychiatric Association, Philadelphia, Nov. 20 (II B 6; II C 1).

Fernandez-Zoila, A., & Lebreton, M. (1958), Social distance and interpersonal relations in psychiatric setting: Technical aspects of psychosocial approach. *Ann. Med. Psychol. Paris*, 116:224-254 (French) (I B 1).

Ferndale, J. (1963), *The Day Hospital Movement in Great Britain.* N.Y., Oxford, Paris: Pergamon Press (II B 5).

Field, M. (1955), The nurse and the social worker on the hospital team. *Amer. J. Nurs.*, 55:694-696 (II A 3 g; II A 3 f).

Fields, J. F. (1960), Putting theory into practice. *Amer. J. Nurs.*, 60:1294-1295 (II A 3 g; I C 3).

Fink. P. J., & Zerof, H. (1971), Mental health technology: An approach to the manpower problem. *Amer J. Psychiat.*, 127:1082-1085 (I C 1).

Fisher, S., & Morton, R. B. (1957), An exploratory study of some relationships between hospital ward structures and attitudes of ward personnel. *J. Psychol.*, 44:155-164 (I B 1).

Fisher, S. H., & Beard, J. H. (1962), Fountain House: A psychiatric rehabilitation program. In: Masserman, J. H. (Ed.), *Current Psychiatric Therapies*, 2:211-218. N.Y.: Grune & Stratton (II B 5; II B 3).

Fitzsimmons, L. W. (1950), What a nurse looks for in the administrator. *Amer. J. Psychiat.*, 107-173 (II A 3 g; II A 3 b; I B 2; I B 3).

Flamm, G. H. (Mod.) (1975), Hospital psychiatry: Network, web, or maze? Presented to the Annual Meeting of the American Psychiatric Association, Anaheim, Calif., May 5-9. *Scientific Proceedings in Summary Form.* Wash., D.C.: Amer. Psychiat. Assoc., p. 319 (I C 3).

Fleck, S. (1962), Psychiatric hospitalization as a family experience. *Forest Hosp. Publ.*, 1:29-37 (II B 4).

—— (1963), Psychotherapy of families of hospitalized patients. In: Masserman, J. H. (Ed.), *Current Psychiatric Therapies* 3:211-218. N.Y.: Grune & Stratton (II B 4).

——, Cornelison, A. R., Norton, L., & Lidz, T. (1957), Interaction between hospital staff and families. *Psychiatry*, 20:343-350 (II B 4).

Fleming, J., & Hamburg, D. A. (1958), An analysis of methods for teaching psychotherapy with description of a new approach. *AMA Arch. Neurol. & Psychiat.* 79:179-200 (II C 1).

Folkard, S. (1960), Aggressive behavior in relation to open wards in mental hospitals. *Ment. Hygiene,* 44:155-161 (II B 2; II B 3).

Folsom, G. S. (1963), The music therapists' special contributions. *Ment. Hosp.,* 14:638-642 (II A 3 h; II A 2).

Forman, J. (1951), The therapeutic team: A consideration of the collective collaborative roles of doctor, nurse, attendant and family. *Ohio Med. J.,* 47:321-325 (II A 2; II A 3; I B 3; II B 4).

Forstenzer, H. M. (1961), Problems in relating community programs to state hospitals. *Amer. J. Public Health,* 51:1152-1157 (II B 6; I A 2).

Fox, P. D., & Rappaport, M. (1972), Some approaches to evaluating community mental health services. *Arch. Gen Psychiat.,* 26: 172-178 (II B 7).

Framo, J. L., & Adlerstein, A. M. (1961), A behavioral disturbance index for psychiatric patient and ward disturbance. *J. Clin. Psychol.,* 17:260-264 (II C 2; I B 1).

Frank, M. H. (1949), Volunteer work with psychiatric patients. *Ment. Hygiene,* 33:353-365 (II A 3 j).

Freeman, H. E., & Simmons, O. G. (1958), Wives, mothers, and the post-hospital performance of mental patients. *Soc. Forces,* 37:153-159 (II B 4; II B 5).

Freeman, T. (1960), The psychoanalyst in the mental hospital. *Brit. J. Med. Psychol.,* 33:279-282 (II A 3 b; I C 3; II C 1).

Freudenthal, K. (1949), Participation of the community agency in hospital discharge planning. *J. Soc. Casework,* 30:421-426 (II B 6; II B 5).

Friedman, J. H. (1963), An organization of ex-patients for follow-up therapy. In: Masserman, J. H. (Ed.), *Current Psychiatric Therapies,* 3:272-276. N.Y.: Grune & Stratton (II B 3; II B 5).

Fryling, V. B., & Fryling, A. G. (1960), Patients' attitudes toward socio-therapy. *Psychiat. Quart.,* 34:97-115 (II B 1; I B 1; II B 3).

Fuller, R. G. (1954), A study of administration of state psychiatric services. *Ment. Hygiene,* 38:177 (I B 2).

Gaede, D. C. (1962), The private hospital. In symbiosis with state institutions. *Ment. Hosp.,* 13:487-488 (II B 6; II C 1; I C 1; I A 2).

Gaitonde, M. R. (1963), Clinical psychiatric training. Psychiatric clinical clerkship at the University of Kansas Medical Center. *J. Kansas Med. Soc.,* 64:93-100 (II C 1).

Galioni, E. G. (1952), Report of Stockton pilot study July 1, 1950-Dec. 31, 1951. Sacramento, Calif.: Calif. Dept. Ment Hygiene (II A 3; I C 3; II B 1; II B 3).

―――― (1960), Evaluation of a treatment program for chronically ill schizophrenic patients―a six year program. In: Appleby, L., Scher, J. M., & Cummings, J. (Eds.), *Chronic Schizophrenia*. Glencoe, Ill.: Free Press, pp. 303-324 (I C 3).

――――, Adams, F. H., & Tallman, F. F. (1953), Intensive treatment of backward patients―a controlled pilot study. *Amer. J. Psychiat.*, 109:576-583 (II A 3; I C 3; II B 1; II B 3).

――――, Notman, R. R., Stanton, A. H., & Williams, R. H. (1957), The nature and purposes of mental hospital wards. In: Greenblatt, M., Levinson, D. J., & Wiliams, R. H. (Eds.) (1957), pp. 327-356 (I B 1; I C 3; II B 1).

Gallagher, E. B., & Albert, R. S. (1961), The Gelbdorf affair; an examination of institutional dilemmas in a progressive mental hospital. *Psychiatry*, 24:221-227 (I B 1).

――――, Sharaf, M. R., & Levinson, D. J. (1965), The influence of patient and therapist in determining the use of psychotherapy in a hospital setting. *Psychiatry*, 28:297-310 (I C 3).

Gammon, R. (1950), *A Survey of the Mental Institutions of South State*. Wash., D.C.: U.S. Public Health Serv. (I A 1).

Garber, R. S. (1958), Legal implications of the open hospital. *Ment. Hosp.*, 9:24-25 (II B 2; I B 2).

―――― (1963), The hospital, the family doctor, and aftercare. *Ment. Hosp.*, 14:214-215 (II B 5; II B 6).

―――― (1964), Administrative principles as adjuncts to therapy. *Ment. Hosp.*, 15:400-401 (I B 2; I C 3; I B 1).

Garcia, L. B. (1960), The Clarinda plan: An ecological approach to hospital organization. *Ment. Hosp.*, 11:30-31 (I B 2; I C 3).

Gardner, E. A. (1968), Indigenous persons as clinic therapists in a community mental health center; implications for new careers. Presented to the Annual Meeting of the American Psychiatric Association, Boston, May 13-17 (II B 7).

Gardner, G. (1950), Contribution of the present-day psychologist to the clinical team. In: *Education for Psychiatric Social Workers*. N.Y.: Amer. Assoc. Psychiat. Soc. Workers, pp. 41-54 (II A 3 e; II A 2).

Gartenberg, G. (1959), Developing procedural manuals for institutions. *Ment. Hosp.*, 10:35-36 (I B 2; I C 3).

Garza-Guerrero, A. C. (1975), Therapeutic use of social subsystems in a hospital setting. *J. Nat. Assoc. Priv. Psychiat. Hosp.*, 7:23-29 (II B 1).

Geller, J. J., Chlenoff, S., & Goldman, A. (1964), Basic shift in staff-patient relationships in a large mental hospital. Presented to the Annual Meeting of the American Psychiatric Association, Los Angeles, May 7 (I B 1).

Gerjuoy, H., Rosenberg, B. G., Bond, J. G., McDevitt, R., & Balogh, J. K. (1963), Mental hospital ward attendants' work attitudes and their work experience in "front" or "back" wards. *J. Gen. Psychol.*, 68:173-180 (II A 3 i).

Gerty, F. J. (1963), The role of the state in the care of the mentally ill. *Proc. Inst. Med. Chicago*, 24:249-251 (I A 1; I C 3).

_____ (1964), Roles and responsibilities in mental health planning. Presented to the Annual Meeting of the American Psychiatric Association, Los Angeles, May 8 (II B 6).

Gertz, B. (1963), *Human Relations Training with Mental Hospital Personnel—A Report on Laboratory Training.* Columbia, S.C.: South Carolina State Hosp. (I B 3; II C 1).

Gilbert, D. C. (1954) Ideologies concerning mental illness: A socio-psychological study of mental hospital personnel. Cambridge, Mass.: Unpublished doctoral dissertation, Radcliffe College (I B 1; II A 3 a).

_____ & Levinson, D. J. (1956), Ideology, personality and institutional policy in the mental hospital. *J. Abn. & Soc. Psychol.*, 53:263-271 (I B 1; I B 2).

_____ _____ (1957a), "Custodialism" and "humanism" in mental hospital structure and in staff ideology. In: Greenblatt, M., Levinson, D. J., & Williams, R. H. (Eds.) (1957), pp. 20-35. Revised in *J. Abn. & Soc. Psychol.*, 53:263-271 (I B 1; I C 3).

_____ _____ (1957b), Role performance, ideology, and personality in mental hospital aides. In: Greenblatt, M., Levinson, D. J., & Williams, R. H. (Eds.) (1957), pp. 197-208, (II A 3 i; I B 1).

Gilbert, J. E. (1959), The open door philosophy: Reflections from the past. *Med. Serv. J. Canada*, 15:545-550 (II B 2).

Glasscote, R. M. (1971), The mental health center: Portents and prospects. *Amer. J. Psychiat.*, 127:940-941 (II B 7).

_____ , Kraft, A. M., Glassman, S. M., & Jepson, W. W. (1969), *Partial Hospitalization for the Mentally Ill: A Study of Programs and Problems.* Wash., D.C.: Joint Info. Serv. of Amer. Psychiat. Assoc. & Nat. Assoc. Ment. Health (II B 5).

_____ , Sanders, D., Forstenzer, H. M., & Foley, A. R. (1964), *The Community Mental Health Center—An Analysis of Existing Models.* Wash., D.C.: Amer. Psychiat. Assoc. (II B 7).

————— , Sussex, J. N., Cummings, E., et al. (1969), *The Community Mental Health Center—An Interim Appraisal.* Wash., D.C.: Joint Info. Serv. of Amer. Psychiat. Assoc. & Nat. Assoc. Ment. Health (II B 7).

Glick, I. D. (Mod.) (1975), Controlled studies of alternative lengths of hospitalization for psychiatric illness. Presented to the Annual Meeting of the American Psychiatric Association, Anaheim, Calif., May 5-9. *Scientific Proceedings in Summary Form.* Wash., D.C.: Amer. Psychiat. Assoc., p. 325 (II C 2).

————— , Hargreaves, W. A., Dures, J., & Showstack, J. (1975), Short *vs.* long hospitalization: One year follow-up. Presented to the Annual Meeting of the American Psychiatric Association, Anaheim, Calif., May 5-9, *Scientific Proceedings in Summary Form.* Wash., D.C.: Amer. Psychiat. Assoc., pp. 219-220 (I C 2).

Gluckmann, R. (1955), The chaplain as a member of a diagnostic clinical team. *Ment. Hygiene,* 37:278 (II A 3 k; II A 2).

Glueck, B. C., Jr. (1963), Research in mental hospitals. *Ment. Hosp.,* 14:93-97 (II C 2).

Goffman, E. (1957), On the characteristics of total institutions. In: *Symposium on Preventive and Social Psychiatry.* Wash., D.C.: Walter Reed Army Institute of Research, pp. 43-84. Longer version in: Goffman, E. (1961), pp. 3-124 (II B 6; I B 1).

————— (1959), The moral career of the mental patient. *Psychiatry,* 22:123-142. Also in: Goffman, E. (1961), pp. 125-170 (I B 1; I C 3; II B 3).

————— (1961), *Asylums—Essays on the Social Situation of Mental Patients and Other Inmates.* Chicago: Aldine (I B 1; I C 3; I B 2; I C 2).

Goldberg, A., & Rubin, B. (1964), Recovery of patients during periods of supposed neglect. *Brit. J. Med. Psychol.,* 37:265-272 (I A 1; I C 1; I C 3).

Goldberg, D. (1971), The scope and limits of community psychiatry. In: Shagass, C. (Ed.), *Modern Problems of Pharmacopsychiatry,* 6:5-25. Basel: Karger (II B 7).

Goldberg, N., & Hyde, R. W. (1954), Role-playing in psychiatric training. *J. Soc. Psychol.,* 39:63-75 (II C 1).

Goldman, A. E., & Lawton, M. P. (1962), The role of the psychiatric aide: A report of the Norristown seminar. *Ment. Hygiene,* 48:288-298 (II A 3 i).

Gooddy, W., Gautier-Smith, P. C., & Dunkley, P. W. (1960),

Neurological practice in a mental observation unit. *Lancet,* 2:1290-1292 (II A 3 d).

Gordon, H. L., & Groth, C. (1961), Mental patients wanting to stay in the hospital. *Arch. Gen. Psychiat.,* 4:124-130 (I C 3).

Gore, C. P., & Jones, K. (1961), Survey of long-stay mental hospital population. *Lancet,* 2:544-546 (I A 1).

Gorman, M. (1963), Mental health care. Striking changes ahead. *Hosp. Manag.,* 96:61-63 (I A 1; I C 3).

Goshen, C. E. (1961), Current status of mental health manpower. *Arch. Gen. Psychiat.,* 5:266-275 (I C 1; I A 1).

Graham, E. C., & Mullen, M. M. (1956), *Rehabilitation Literature, 1950-1955.* N.Y.: McGraw-Hill (II A 3 h; I C 3).

Graham, E. M. (1964), Group programs for nursing service personnel in psychiatric hospitals. Presented to the Annual Meeting of the American Psychiatric Association, Los Angeles, May 8 (II A 3 g; I C 3).

Graham, T. G., & Zingery, J. W. (1961), Turnover of psychiatric attendants. *J. Clin. Exp. Psychopath.,* 22:95-105 (II A 3 i; I C 1).

Gralnick, A. (ed.) (1969), *The Psychiatric Hospital as a Therapeutic Instrument: Collected Papers of High Point Hospital.* N.Y.: Brunner/Mazel (I C 3).

_____ (Ed.) (1975), *Humanizing the Psychiatric Hospital.* N.Y.: Jason Aronson (I C 3).

_____ & D'Elia, F. (1961), Role of the patient in the therapeutic community: Patient-participation. *Amer. J. Psychother.,* 15: 63-72 (II B 3; II B 1).

Gray, J. R. (1968), *The Comprehensive Community Mental Health Center and Continuity of Care.* Chapel Hill, N.C.: School of Public Health, Univ. North Carolina (II B 7).

Greco, J. T. (1961), Two roads to treatment. II. The case for the psychiatric unit. *Ment. Hosp.,* 12:10-12 (II A 1; I C 3).

Greenblatt, M. (1957a), The movement from custodial hospital to therapeutic community: Implications for psychiatry and hospital practice. In: Greenblatt, M., Levinson, D. J., & Williams, R. H. (Eds.) (1957), pp. 611-619 (I C 3; II B 1; II C 1; II B 3; II B 5; II B 6).

_____ (1957b), The psychiatrist as social system clinician. In: Greenblatt, M., Levinson, D. J., & Williams, R. H. (Eds.) (1957), pp. 317-323 (II A 3 c; I B 1).

_____ (1958), Research and demonstration of value of combined hospital-patient-community participation in rehabilitation of the mentally ill. In: *An Inventory of Social and Economic Research in Health.* N.Y.: Health Info. Found., pp. 93-95 (II B 6; II B 5; II C 2).

———— (1962), Conducting a research department. *Ment. Hosp.,* 13:580-581 (II C 2).

———— (1963), Beyond the therapeutic community. *J. Hillside Hosp.,* 12: Nos. 3 & 4 (II B 1).

———— (1975), Phase-out of mental hospitals in America. Presented to the Annual Meeting of the American Psychiatric Association, Anaheim, Calif., May 5-9. *Scientific Proceedings in Summary Form.* Wash., D.C.: Amer. Psychiat. Assoc., pp. 218-219 (I A 1).

———— & Levinson, D. H. (1959), Issues in therapeutic organization. *Psychiat. Res. Rep., Amer. Psychiat. Assoc.,* 11:13-29 (II B 1; I B 2; I C 3).

————, ———— & Williams, R. H. (Eds.) (1957), *The Patient and the Mental Hospital.* Glencoe, Ill.: Free Press (I B 1; I C 3; II B 1; II C 1; I B 2; II C 2).

———— & Lidz, T. (1957), The patient and the extra-hospital world; some dimensions of the problem. In: Greenblatt, M., Levinson, D. J., & Williams, R. H. (Eds.) (1957), pp. 501-516 (II B 2; II B 5; II B 6).

————, Moore, R. F., Albert, R. S., & Soloman, M. H. (1963), *The Prevention of Hospitalization—Treatment without Admission for Psychiatric Patients.* N.Y.: Grune & Stratton (II B 5; II B 6).

———— , Solomon, M., Evans, A. S., & Brooks, G. W. (Eds.) (1965), *Drug and Social Therapy in Chronic Schizophrenia.* Springfield, Ill.: Charles C Thomas (I C 3; II B 1).

————, York, R., Brown, E. L., & Hyde, R. W. (1955), *From Custodial to Therapeutic Care in Mental Hospitals.* N.Y.: Russell Sage Found. (I C 3).

Greenhill, M., Gralnick, A., Duncan, R., Yemez, R., & Turker, F. (1966), Considerations in evaluating the results of psychotherapy with 500 inpatients. *Amer. J. Psychother.,* 20:58 (I C 3).

Grimes, J. M. (1951), *When Minds Go Wrong.* Chicago: published privately by the author (I A 1; I C 3).

———— (1954), *When Minds Go Wrong—The Truth About Our Mentally Ill and Their Care in Mental Hospitals.* N.Y.: Devon-Adair (I A 1; I C 3).

Grob, G. (1966), *The State and the Mentally Ill.* Chapel Hill, N.C.: Univ. of North Carolina Press (I A 1).

_____ (1973), *Mental Institutions in America.* N.Y.: Free Press (I A 1).

Group for the Advancement of Psychiatry (1948a), The psychiatric social worker in the psychiatric hospital. Report No. 2. Topeka: GAP (II A 3 f).

_____ (1948b), Public psychiatric hospitals. Report No. 5. Topeka: GAP (I A 1; I C 3; I C 1; I A 2).

_____ (1949), Statistics pertinent to psychiatry in the U.S. Report No. 7. Topeka: GAP (I A 1).

_____ (1950), The problem of the aged patient in the public psychiatric hospital. Report No. 14. Topeka: GAP (I A 1; I C 3).

_____ (1952), The psychiatric nurse in the mental hospital. Report No. 22. Topeka: GAP (II A 3 g).

_____ (1953), Outline to be used as a guide to the evaluation of treatment in a public psychiatric hospital. Report No. 23. Topeka: GAP (I C 3; I B 2; I A 1).

_____ (1954), Collaborative research in psychopathology. Report No. 25. N.Y.: GAP (II C 2; II A 2).

_____ (1955), Therapeutic use of the self—a concept for teaching patient care. Report No. 33. Topeka: GAP (II A 3 g; II C 1; I C 3).

_____ (1961a), Administration of the public psychiatric hospital. Report No. 46. N.Y.: GAP (I B 2).

_____ (1961b), Toward therapeutic care. A guide for those who work with the mentally ill. Report No. 51. N.Y.: GAP (II A 3; I C 3).

_____ (1961c), Problems in estimating changes in frequency of mental disorders. Report No. 50. N.Y.: GAP (I A 1).

_____ (1963), Public relations: A responsibility of the mental hospital administrator. Report No. 55. N.Y.: GAP (II B 6; I B 2).

_____ (1964), Urban America and the planning of mental health services. Symposium No. 10. N.Y.: GAP (I A 1; II B 6).

_____ (1969), Crisis in psychiatric hospitalization. Report No. 72. Topeka: GAP (I A 1).

Gurel, L. (Ed.) (1964), Intramural report, 1964-5: An assessment of psychiatric hospital effectiveness. Wash., D.C.: V.A. Psychiat. Eval. Project (I A 1).

Gussen, J. (1960), An experimental day-night hospital. *Ment. Hosp.,* 11:26-29 (II B 5).

Gynther, M. D., & Gall, H. S. (1964), Therapeutic community: Concept, practice and evaluation. In: Wessen, A. F. (1964), pp. 169-175 (II B 1).

———, Reznikoff, M., & Fishman, M. (1963), Attitudes of psychiatric patients toward treatment, psychiatrists and mental hospitals. *J. Nerv. Ment. Dis.*, 136:68-71 (II B 3; II A 3 c; I B 1).

Hacken, E., & Hunt, R. C. (1959), Open ward management of acute patients in a multi-story building. *Psychiat. Quart.* (Suppl.), 33:89-96 (II B 2).

Haddock, J. N., & Dundan, H. D. (1951), Volunteer work in a state hospital by college students. *Ment. Hygiene,* 35:599-603 (II A 3 j).

Hagopian, P. B. (1963), Using mental patients as emergency manpower. *Hospitals,* 37:52-53 (II B 3; I C 1).

Hall, B. H. (1948), The psychiatric team. *Psychiat. Aide,* 5:5-6 (II A 2).

——— (1957), Vicissitudes of psychiatric ward personnel. In: Greenblatt, M., Levinson, D. J., & Williams, R. H. (Eds.) (1957), pp. 231-236 (II A 3 i).

——— (1962), Crises and trends in hospital psychiatry. *Hosp. Progr.,* 43:82-87 (I A 1; I C 3).

———, Gangemi, M., Norris, V. L., Vail, V. H., & Sawatsky, G. (1952), *Psychiatric Aide Education.* N.Y.: Grune & Stratton (II A 3 i; II C 1).

Ham, G. C. (1961), The teaching potential of a non-teaching hospital. *J. Med. Educ.,* 36:17-22 (II C 1; I A 2; I C 1).

Hamburg, D. A. (1957), Therapeutic aspects of communication and administrative policy in the psychiatric section of a general hospital. In: Greenblatt, M., Levinson, D. J., & Williams, R. H. (Eds.) (1957), pp. 91-107 (I B 2; I B 3; I B 1; I C 3).

Hamilton, D. M. (1946), The psychiatric hospital as a cultural pattern. In: Glueck, B. (Ed.), *Current Therapies of Personality Disorder.* N.Y.: Grune & Stratton (I B 1).

Hamilton, S. W. (1944), The history of American mental hospitals. In: *One-Hundred Years of American Psychiatry.* N.Y.: Columbia Univ. Press (I A 1; I C 3).

Hammersley, D. W., & Hart, G. (1963), *Opinions of Selected Mental Health Authorities Regarding the Usefulness of a National Service Corps.* Wash., D.C.: Amer. Psychiat. Assoc., Ment. Hosp. Serv. (II A 3).

——— & Vosburgh, P. (1967), Iowa's shrinking mental hospital population. *Hosp. & Commun. Psychiat.,* 18:106-116 (I A 1).

Hanlon, J. G. (1961), Social Service responsibilities in a state hospital. *Virginia Med. Monthly,* 88:105-110 (II A 3 f).

Hansell, N. (1968), Casualty management method. *Arch. Gen. Psychiat.,* 19:281-289 (II B 7).

_____ & Hart, D. W. (1970), Local service growth: The Illinois zone plan. *Amer. J. Psychiat.*, 127:686-690 (I A 2; I A 1).

Hargreaves, A., Warsaw, P., & Lewis, E. (1962), Day hospital for psychiatric patients. *Amer. J. Nurs.*, 62:80-85 (II B 5).

Harlow, M., Jones, D., Roberts, W., Thompson, P., & Wheeler, F. (1956), The therapeutic environment provided through a multidisciplinary approach. In: *Group Work in a Psychiatric Setting*. N.Y.: Whiteside (II A 2; II B 1; I C 3).

Harris, P., & Johnson, R. W. (1961), Recognition and development of aides' potentials. *Ment. Hosp.*, 12:26-27 (II A 3 i; II C 1).

Harrower, M. (Ed.) (1955), *Medical and Psychological Team Work in the Care of the Chronically Ill*. Springfield, Ill.: Charles C Thomas (II A 2; I C 3).

Hart, W. T., & Bassett, L. (1972), Delivery of services to lower socioeconomic groups by a suburban community mental health center. *Amer. J. Psychiat.*, 129:191-196 (II B 7).

Harvey, B., & Monk, R. (1958), Sociogramatic study of spontaneous patient groupings. *Canad. Nurse*, 54:924-928 (I B 1; II B 3).

Harwood, J. A. (1960), Social services on a continued treatment ward. *Ment. Hosp.*, 11:7-11 (II A 3 f; I C 3).

Haun, P. (1950), Psychiatry and the ancillary services. *Amer. J. Psychiat.*, 107:102-109 (II A 3).

Hawkins, D. M., Norton, C. B., Eisdorfer, C., & Gianturco, D. (1973), Group process research: A factor analytical study. *Amer. J. Psychiat.*, 130:916-919 (II B 1).

Hawkins, N. G. (1961), A research program for a state mental hospital (Hollidayberg) in Pennsylvania: A critical review of the pertinent literature. *J. Amer. Geriat. Soc.*, 9:523-276 (II C 2).

_____ (1963), Mental hospitals as political machines. *Med. Times*, 91:536-546 (I B 1; II B 6).

Hayes, J. L. (1959), A layman's view of hospital leadership. *Ment. Hosp.*, 10:43-46 (I B 1; I B 2; I C 2).

Haythorn, W., Couch, A., Haefner, P., Langham, P., & Carter, L. (1956), The behavior of authoritarian and equalitarian personalities in groups. *Human Relations*, 9:57-74 (I B 3; I B 1; I B 2; I C 2).

Hayward, S. T. (1963), On being ill in a mental hospital. *Brit. J. Med. Psychol.*, 36:57-65 (II B 3).

Heninger, O. P. (1963), The process of decentralization at the Utah State Hospital. *Provo Papers*, 7:1-18. Presented originally to

"The Unit Plan Conference," Norristown State Hospital, Norristown, Pa., Feb. 25 (II A 1; I B 2).

Henry, J. (1954), The formal social structure of a psychiatric hospital. *Psychiatry*, 17:139-151 (I B 1; I B 2; I C 2).

―――― (1957), Types of institutional structure. In: Greenblatt, M., Levinson, D. J., & Williams, R. H. (Eds.) (1957), pp. 73-90 (I B 1; I B 2; I C 2).

―――― (1964), Space and power on a psychiatric unit. In: Wesson, A. F. (1964), pp. 20-34 (I B 1; II A 1; I B 2; I C 2).

Herz, M. I. (1972), The therapeutic community: A critique. *Hosp. & Commun. Psychiat.*, 23 (II B 1).

―――― , Endicott, J., & Spitzer, R. L. (1975), Brief *vs.* standard hospitalization: The families. Presented to the Annual Meeting of the American Psychiatric Association, Anaheim, Calif., May 5-9. *Scientific Proceedings in Summary Form.* Wash., D.C.: Amer. Psychiat. Assoc., pp. 22-23 (I C 3; II B 4).

Hes, J. P., & Handler, S. L. (1961), Multidimensional group psychotherapy. *Arch. Gen. Psychiat.*, 5:70-75 (II B 1).

Hjelholt, G., & Miles, M. B. (1963), Extending the conventional training laboratory design. *J. Amer. Soc. Training Directors.* Wash., D.C.: Nat. Training Labs.-Nat. Educ. Assoc., Subscrip. Serv. No. 1 (I B 3).

Hobbs, G. E., Wanklin, J., & Ladd, K. B. (1965), Changing patterns of mental hospital discharges and readmissions in the past two decades. *Canad. Med. Assoc. J.*, 93:17-20 (I A 1).

Hoch, P. H., & Rado, S. (1961), A graduate school for psychiatric education of physicians in mental hospital service. *Amer. J. Psychiat.*, 117:883-886 (II C 1; I A 2; I C 1).

Hoffman, J. L. (1957), Problems of administration in a large mental hospital. In: Greenblatt, M., Levinson, D. J., & Williams, R. H. (Eds.) (1957), pp. 46-48 (I B 2).

Hogarty, G. E., & Ulrich, R. (1972), The discharge readiness inventory. *Arch. Gen. Psychiat.*, 26:419-426 (I C 3).

Hollingshead, A. B., & Redlich, F. C. (1958), *Social Class and Mental Illness.* N.Y.: Wiley (I A 1; I C 3).

Holzberg, J. D. (1960), Problems in the team treatment of adults in state mental hospitals. Panel, 1958. I. The historical traditions of the state hospital as a force of resistance to the team. *Amer. J. Orthopsychiat.*, 30:87-94 (I B 3; II A 2; I C 3; I A 1; I B 1).

Horwitz, L. (1968), Group psychotherapy training for psychiatric residents. *Curr. Psychiat. Ther.*, 8:223-233 (II B 1; II C 1).

Houck, J. H. (1975), The future of the private psychiatric hospital. *Psychiat. Ann.,* 5:25-36 (I A 1).

Howard, A. R. (1959), The patient speaks: Inter-patient relations. *Ment. Hosp.,* 10(6):26 (II B 3).

Hunt, R. C. (1960), The state hospital stereotype. *Ment. Hosp.,* 11: 17-18 (I B 3; I C 1; I A 1).

———, Gruenberg, E. M., Hacker, E., & Huxley, M. (1961), A comprehensive hospital-community service in a state hospital. *Amer. J. Psychiat.,* 17:817-821 (II B 6).

Hunter, R. A. (1956), The rise and fall of mental nursing. *Lancet,* 1:98-99 (II A 3 g).

Hurd, H. M., Drewry, W. F., Dewey, R., Pilgrim, C. W., Bulmer, G.A., & Burgess, T. J. W. (Eds.) (1916), *The Institutional Care of the Insane in the United States and Canada,* Vol. III. Baltimore: Johns Hopkins Press (I A 1; I C 3).

Hurst, L. C. (1957), The unlocking of wards in mental hospitals. *Amer. J. Psychiat.,* 114:306-308 (II B 2).

Hutchinson, J. T. (1963), Psychiatry and medical administration. *Lancet,* 1:1314-1315 (I B 2; I C 3).

Hutt, M. L., Menninger, W. C., & O'Keefe, D. E. (1947), The neuropsychiatric team in the U.S. Army. *Ment. Hygiene,* 31: 103-119 (II A 2; II C 3).

Hyde, R. W. (1955), *Experiencing the Patient's Day: A Manual for Psychiatric Hospital Personnel.* N.Y.: Putnam (II A 3; II B 3).

———, Greenblatt, M., & Wells, F. L. (1956), The role of the attendant in authority and compliance: Notes on ten cases. *J. Gen. Psychol.,* 54:107-126 (II A 3 i; I B 2; I C 2; I B 1).

——— & Solomon, H. C. (1950), Patient government; a new form of group therapy. *Digest Neurol. & Psychiat.,* 18:207-218 (II B 3; I C 3).

——— ——— (1951), Clinical management of psychiatric hospitals. *Connecticut Med. J.,* 15:391-398 (I C 2; I B 2).

——— & Williams, R. H. (1957), What is therapy and who does it? In: Greenblatt, M., Levinson, D. J., & Williams, R. H. (Eds.) (1957), pp. 173-196 (II A 3; I C 3).

Imre, P. D. (1962), Attitudes of volunteers toward mental hospitals compared to patients and personnel. *J. Clin. Psychol.,* 18:516 (I B 1; II A 3 i; II B 3).

——— & Wolf, S. (1962), Attitudes of patients and personnel toward mental hospitals. *J. Clin. Psychol.,* 18:232-234 (I B 1; II B 3).

Irwin, T. D. (1963), An activity-centered resocialization program. *Ment. Hosp.,* 14:405-406 (II A 3 h; I C 3; II B 1).

Ishiyama, T., & Grover, W. L. (1960), The phenomenon of resistance to change in a large psychiatric institution. *Psychiat. Quart.,* 34:1-11 (I B 1; I B 2).

Jackson, D. D., & Weakland, J. H. (1961), Conjoint family therapy. *Psychiatry,* 24:30-45 (II B 4).

Jackson, J. (1964), Toward a comparative study of mental hospitals: Characteristics of the treatment environment. In: Wessen, A. F. (1964), pp. 35-90 (I C 3; II B 1; I A 1; I B 1).

Jacoby, M. G. (1959), Patient government. *Amer. J. Psychiat.* 115:943-944 (II B 3).

———— & McLamb, E. C. (1959), Adjusting to permissiveness in a state hospital. *Amer. J. Nurs.,* 59:1742-1743 (II B 1; I C 3; I B 1).

Jacques, E. (1948), Interpretive group discussion as a method of facilitating social change. A progress report on the use of group methods in the investigation and resolution of social problems. *Human Relations,* 1:533-549 (I B 3; I B 2; II B 1).

———— (1953), On the dynamics of social structure. *Human Relations,* 6:3-24 (I B 1).

———— (1955), Social systems as a defense against persecutory and depressive anxiety. In: Klein, M., Heinmann, P., & Money-Kyrle, E. (Eds.), *New Directions in Psychoanalysis.* London: Tavistock, pp. 478-498 (I B 1).

———— (1957), Some principles of organization of a social therapeutic institution. *J. Soc. Issues,* 3:4-10 (I B 1; II B 1; I C 3).

Jaffary, S. K. (1942), *The Mentally Ill and Public Provision for Their Care in Illinois.* Chicago: Univ. of Chicago Press (I A 1; I C 3).

Johnson, D. M., & Dodds, N. (1957), *The Plea for the Silent.* London: Christopher Johnson (I A 1; I C 3).

Johnson, M., & Whitney, O. P. (1962), In-service education for psychiatric aides. *Ment. Hosp.,* 13:31-34 (II A 3 i; II C 1).

Joint Commission on Mental Illness and Health (1961), *Action for Mental Health.* N.Y.: Basic Books (I A 1; I C 3).

Joint Information Service of the American Psychiatric Association and the National Association for Mental Health (1960), *Fifteen Indices—An Aid in Reviewing State Mental Health and Hospital Programs.* Wash., D.C.: Amer. Psychiat. Assoc. (I A 1; I C 3).

Jones, G. L., & Waldrum, A. F. (1960), Present-day concepts in nursing service administration in hospitals for the mentally ill. *Amer. J. Psychiat.,* 117:329-335 (II A 3 g; I B 2).

Jones, K. (1955), *Lunacy, Law, and Conscience.* London: Routledge & Kegan Paul (I A 1; I C 3).

———— , Sidebotham, R., Wadsworth, W. V., Torge, W. L., & Price, H. M. (1961), Cost and efficiency in mental hospitals. *Hospital* (London), 57:23-25 (I A 1).

Jones, M. (1952a), *Social Psychiatry*. London: Tavistock (II B 1; I C 3; I B 1).

———— (1952b), *Rehabilitation*. Geneva: World Health Org. (I C 3; II B 1; II B 3; II A 3 h).

———— (1953), *The Therapeutic Community*. N.Y.: Basic Books (II B 1).

———— (1956), The concept of a therapeutic community. *Amer. J. Psychiat.*, 112:647 (II B 1).

———— (1961), Community aspects of hospital treatment. *Curr. Psychiat. Ther.*, 1:196-203 (II B 6).

———— (1962), Settings for treatment and training in social psychiatry. *Ment. Hosp.*, 13:646-650 (II C 1; I C 3; II B 1; I B 1).

———— (1968a), *Beyond the Therapeutic Community*. New Haven: Yale University Press (II B 1).

———— (1968b), *Social Psychiatry in Practice*. Baltimore: Pelican Penguin Books (II B 1).

———— (1973), Therapeutic milieu *versus* professional and institutional conservatism. *Roche Report, Frontiers of Psychiatry*, 3:1-2 (II B 1).

———— & Matthews, R. A. (1956), The application of the therapeutic community principle to a state mental hospital program. *Brit. J. Med. Psychol.*, 29:57-62 (II B 1).

———— & Rapoport, R. (1955), Administrative and social psychiatry. *Lancet*, 2:386-388 (II B 1; I B 2; I B 1).

———— ———— (1957), The absorption of new doctors into a therapeutic community. In: Greenblatt, M., Levinson, D. J., & Williams, R. H. (Eds.) (1957), pp. 248-262 (II B 1; I B 3; I C 2).

———— & Tuxford, J. (1963), Some common trends in British and American mental hospital psychiatry. *Lancet*, 1:433-435 (II B 1; I C 3; I A 1; I B 2).

Jones, N. F., Kahn, M. W., & MacDonald, J. M. (1963), Psychiatric patients' views of mental illness, hospitalization and treatment. *J. Nerv. Ment. Dis.*, 136:82-87 (II B 3; I C 3; I B 1).

Jones, R. O. (1958), New perspectives in hospital and community relations. *Ment. Hosp.*, 9:6-14 (II B 6).

Kahn, J. P. (1959), The role of ancillary personnel in the total treatment of psychiatric patients. *Ment. Hosp.*, 10(6):27 (II A 3 a; I C 3).

Kahn, M. W., Jones, N. F., MacDonald, J. M., Conners, C. K., & Burchard, J. (1963), A factorial study of patient attitudes toward mental illness and psychiatric hospitalization. *J. Clin. Psychol.*, 19:235-241 (II B 3; I C 3; II C 2).

Kahn, R. L., Pollack, M., & Fink, M. (1957), Social factors in the selection of therapy in a voluntary mental hospital. *J. Hillside Hosp.*, 6:216-228 (I B 1).

Kahne, M. J. (1959), Democratic structure and impersonal experience in mental hospitals. *Psychiatry*, 22:363-375 (I B 1; I B 2).

Kandel, D. B., & Williams, R. H. (1964), *Psychiatric Rehabilitation: Some Problems of Research.* N.Y.: Atherton (II C 2).

Kanno, C. K., & Scheidemandel, P. L. (1970), *Salary Ranges of Personnel Employed in State Mental Hospitals and Community Mental Health Centers.* Wash., D.C.: Amer. Psychiat. Assoc., Joint Info. Serv. (I A 1; I C 1).

――――, ――――, Glasscote, M. A., & Hammersley, D. (1974), *Psychiatric Treatment in the Community—A National Survey of General Hospital Psychiatric Hospitals.* Wash., D.C.: Amer. Psychiat. Assoc., Joint Info. Serv. (I A 1; II B 7).

Kantor, D. (1957), The use of college students as "case aides" in a social service department of a state hospital: An experiment in undergraduate social work education. In: Greenblatt, M., Levinson, D. J., & Williams, R. H. (Eds.) (1957), pp. 603-608 (II C 1; II A 3 f; II A 3 j).

Kartus, I., & Schlesinger, H. J. (1957), The psychiatric hospital-physician and his patient. In: Greenblatt, M., Levinson, D. J., & Williams, R. H. (Eds.) (1957), pp. 286-299 (II A 3 c; I C 2).

Keeton, J. E. (1964), Goals and pitfalls of day treatment programs. *Ment. Hosp.*, 15:640-643 (II B 5).

Kellam, S. G., & Chassan, J. B. (1962), Social context and symptom fluctuation. *Psychiatry*, 25:370-381 (I B 1).

Kennard, E. A. (1957), Psychiatry, administrative psychiatry, administration: A study of a Veterans Hospital. In: Greenblatt, M., Levinson, D. J., & Williams, R. H. (Eds.) (1957), pp. 36-45 (I B 2; I C 3; I B 1).

Kerkhoff, J. (1952), *How Thin the Veil: A Newspaperman's Story of His Own Crack-up and Recovery.* N.Y.: Greenberg (II B 3; I C 3; I A 1).

Keskiner, A., Zakman, M. J., Rupport, E. H., & Ulett, G. A. (1972), The foster community: A partnership in psychiatric rehabilitation. *Amer. J. Psychiat.*, 129:283-288 (II B 6).

Kessler, D. R. (1964), The structured milieu in the treatment of acute and subacute psychotic reactions. Presented to the Annual Meeting of the American Psychiatric Association, Los Angeles, May 6 (II B 1).

Kidd, H. B. (1961), A team system in a mental hospital. *Lancet*, 2:703-705 (II A 2; II A 1).

Kimbro, C. D., & Lemkau, P. V. (1969), Delays in arranging after-care. *Hosp. & Commun. Psychiat.*, 20:91-92 (II B 5).

Kingston, F. E. (1963), The demand for psychiatric beds. *Lancet*, 1:107-108 (I A 1).

Klemes, M. A. (1951), The therapeutic effect of group morale on a psychiatric hospital ward. *Bull. Menninger Clin.*, 15:58-63 (II B 1; I C 3; I B 1).

Klerman, G. L., & Mallory, V. M. (1963), An integrated male and female clinical service. *Nurs. Outlook*, 11:180-184 (II B 1; I C 3; II B 3).

Klett, C. J., & Lasky, J. J. (1962), Attitudes of staff members toward mental illness and chemotherapy. *Dis. Nerv. Syst.*, 23:101-105 (I B 1).

Klett, S. L., Berger, D. G., Sewall, L. G., & Rice, C. E. (1963), Patient evaluation of the psychiatric wards. *J. Clin. Psychol.*, 19:347-351 (II B 3; I B 1).

Kline, N. S. (1947), *Volunteer Workers*. N.Y.: Nat. Com. Ment. Hygiene (II A 3 j).

———— (1950), Characteristics and screening of unsatisfactory psychiatric attendants and attendant-applicants. *Amer. J. Psychiat.*, 106:569-574 (II A 3 i; I C 1).

Klopfer, W. G., Wylie, A. A., & Hillson, J. S. (1956), Attitudes toward mental hospitals. *J. Clin. Psychol.*, 12:361-365 (II B 6; I B 1).

Kluger, J. M. (1970), The uninsulated caseload in a neighborhood mental health center. *Amer. J. Psychiat.*, 126:1430-1436 (II B 7).

Kolb, L. C. (1962), The metropolis and social psychiatry. *Internat. J. Soc. Psychiat.*, 8:245-249 (II B 6; I B 1).

Koltes, J. (1956), Mental hospitals with open doors. *Amer. J. Psychol.*, 113:250 (II B 2).

Korson, S. M., & Hayes, W. L. (1966), Empathic relationship therapy utilizing student nurses: A five-year pilot study. *Amer. J. Psychiat.*, 123:213-218 (II A 3 g).

Kraft, A., Binner, P., & Dickey, B. (1967), The community mental health program and the longer stay patient. *Arch. Gen. Psychiat.*, 6:64-74 (I C 3; II B 7).

Kramer, B. M. (1962), *Day Hospital (A Study of Partial Hospitalization in Psychiatry)*. N.Y.: Grune & Stratton (II B 5).

Kramer, C. H. (1964), Staff involvement can be overdone. *Ment. Hosp.*, 15:406-408 (I B 3; II B 1).

Kramer, M. (1957), Problems of research on the population dynamics and therapeutic effectiveness of mental hospitals. In: Greenblatt, M., Levinson, D. J., & Williams, R. H. (Eds.) (1957), pp. 145-169 (II C 2; I A 1; I C 3).

———— (1966), Some implications of trends in the usage of psychiatric facilities for community mental health center programs and related research. Wash., D.C.: Public Health Serv. Public. No. 1434, U.S. Govt. Printing Office (II B 7).

———— , Goldstein, H., Israel, R. H., & Johnson, N. A. (1955), *An Historical Study of Disposition of First Admissions to a State Mental Hospital: The Experience of the Warren State Hospital during the Period 1916-50.* Wash., D.C.: Public Health Monogr. No. 32, Pubic Health Serv., Dept. HEW, U.S. Govt. Printing Office (I A 1).

Kraus, P. S. (1957), Ward assignments and patient movement in a large psychiatric hospital. In: Greenblatt, M., Levinson, D. J., & Williams, R. H. (Eds.) (1957), pp. 472-478 (I B 1; I A 1; I C 3).

Kremens, J. B. (1962), A new hospital for modern psychiatry. *Ment. Hosp.*, 13:625-628 (I A 1; I C 3).

Kubie, L. (1968), The future of the private psychiatric hospital. *Internat. J. Psychiat.*, 6:419 (I A 1).

Kurland, A. A. (1962), The Spring Grove State Hospital research program. *Psychopharm. Serv. Cent. Bull.*, 2:87-88 (II C 2).

———— & Nilsson, G. L. (1961), The general practicing physician and the state psychiatric hospital. *Maryland Med. J.*, 10: 134-138 (I A 2; I C 1; II B 6).

Lamb, H. R., & Goertzel, V. (1971), Discharged mental patients — are they really in the community? *Arch. Gen. Psychiat.*, 24: 29-34 (II B 7).

Landy, D. (1961), An anthropological approach to research in the mental hospital community. *Psychiat. Quart.*, 35:741-757 (II C 2; I B 1).

Langsley, D. G., Odland, T. M., Barter, J. T., & Moorehead, W.D. (1973), Who goes to the state hospital now? *Scientific Proceedings in Summary Form.* 126th Annual Meeting of the American Psychiatric Association. Wash., D.C.: Amer. Psychiat. Assoc., p. 231 (I A 1).

Lasky, J. J. (1962), What are some areas for research? In: Gerjuoy, H. (Ed.), *Rehabilitation: Pathways in a Changing World.* Toledo: Univ. Toledo Research Found., pp. 92-102 (II C 2).

Laughlin, H. P. (1954), A group approach to management improvement. *Internat. J. Group Psychother.*, 4:165 (I B 3; I B 2).

Lazarus, J., Locks, B. Z., & Thomas, D. S. (1963), Migration differentials in mental disease state patterns in first admissions to mental hospitals for all disorders and for schizophrenia, New York, Ohio and California, as of 1950. *Milbank Memorial Fund Quart.*, 41:25-42 (I A 1).

Lebar, F. M. (1964), Some implications of ward structure for enculturation of patients. In: Wessen, A. F. (1964), pp. 5-19 (I A 2; I C 3).

Lefebvre, P., Atkins, J., Duckman, J., & Gralnick, A. (1958), The role of the relative in a psychotherapeutic program: Anxiety problems and defensive reactions encountered. *Canad. Psychiat. Assoc. J.*, 3:110-118 (II B 4).

Lefton, M., Dinitz, S., & Pasamanick, B. (1960), Mental hospital organization and staff evaluation of patients. *Arch. Gen. Psychiat.*, 2:462-467 (I B 1; I C 3).

Lehrman, N. S. (1960), A state hospital population five years after admission. *Psychiat. Quart.*, 34:658-681 (I A 1).

Leighton, A. H. (1955), Psychiatric disorder and social environment: An outline for a frame of reference. *Psychiatry*, 18:367-383 (I B 1; II B 1).

_____ (1960), *An Introduction to Social Psychiatry*. Springfield, Ill.: Charles C Thomas (II B 1).

Leipold, W. D., Hoffman, R. F., Bloom, O. J., & Patterson, W. L. (1964), A program for rehumanizing living. *Ment. Hosp.*, 15: 601-602 (II B 1; I B 1; I C 3).

Lemert, E. (1951), *Social Pathology*. N.Y.: McGraw-Hill (II B 1; II B 6; I B 1).

Leopold, R. L. (1967), The west Philadelphia community mental health consortium; administrative planning in a multi-hospital catchment area. *Amer. J. Psychiat.*, 124:69-76 (II B 7).

_____ & Kissick, W. L. (1970), A community mental health center, regional medical program, and joint planning. *Amer. J. Psychiat.*, 126:1718-1726 (II B 7).

Lerner, P. F. (1960), The former patient: A potential volunteer. *Ment. Hosp.*, 11:41 (II A 3 j; II B 3).

Lesser, W. (1955), The team concept—a dynamic factor in treatment. *J. Psychiat. Soc. Work*, 24: 119-126 (II A 2; I C 3).

Letemandia, F. J. J., & Harris, A. D. (1974), Psychiatric services and the future. *Lancet* (Nov. 3):1013-1016 (I A 1).

Levine, J., & Butler, J. (1952), Lecture *vs.* group decision in changing behavior. *J. Appl. Psychol.*, 36:29-33 (I B 3; I B 2).

Levine, M. (1947), Hospitalization as a method of psychotherapy. In: *Psychotherapy in Medical Practice.* N.Y.: Macmillan, p. 65 (I C 3).

Levinson, D. J. (1957), The mental hospital as a research setting: A critical appraisal. In: Greenblatt, M., Levinson, D. J., & Williams, R. H. (Eds.) (1957), pp. 633-649 (II C 2).

———— (1964), *Parenthood in the Mental Hospital.* Boston: Houghton Mifflin (I A 1).

Lewinsohn, P. M., & Nichols, R. C. (1964), The evaluation of changes in psychiatric patients during and after hospitalization. *J. Clin. Psychol.,* 20:272-279 (II C 2).

Lewis, A. B. (1966), Effective utilization of the psychiatric hospital. *JAMA,* 197:871-877 (I C 3).

———— & Selzer, M. (1972), Some neglected issues in milieu therapy. *Hosp. & Commun. Psychiat.,* 23:293-298 (II B 1).

Lewis, G. K. (1960), Report on the seminar project for teachers of psychiatric aides. *Amer. J. Psychiat.,* 117:224-227 (II C 1; II A 3 i).

Leyberg, J. T. (1959), A district psychiatric service: The Bolton pattern. *Lancet,* 2:282-284 (I A 1; II B 6).

Lidz, T., Hotchkiss, G., & Greenblatt, M. (1957), Patient-family-hospital interrelationships: Some general considerations. In: Greenblatt, M., Levinson, D. J., & Williams, R. H. (Eds.) (1957), pp. 535-544 (II B 4).

Lieb, J., Lipsitch, I. I., & Slaby, E. (1973), *The Crisis Team: A Handbook for the Mental Health Professional.* N.Y.: Harper & Row (II A 2).

Lind, A., & Gralnick, A. (1963), Integration of the social group worker and psychiatrist in the psychiatric hospital. Presented to the Annual Meeting of the American Psychiatric Association, St. Louis, May 10 (II A 3 f; II A 3 c; II A 2; I B 3).

Lindsay, J. S. B. (1963), The day hospital and the day patient. *Med. J. Austral.,* 2:777-781 (II B 5).

Linn, L. (1955a), *A Handbook of Hospital Psychiatry—A Practical Guide to Therapy.* N.Y.: Internat. Univ. Press (II C 3; II C 1; I C 3).

———— (1955b), The treatment team. In: Linn, L. (1955a), pp. 113-188 (II A 2).

Lipkin, G. B., & Cohen, R. G. (1973), *Effective Approaches to Patients' Behavior.* N.Y.: Springer (II A 3 g).

Lipsius, S. H. (1973), Judgements of alternatives to hospitalization. *Amer. J. Psychiat.,* 130:892-895 (II B 7).

Liston, M. F. (1960), Psychiatric nursing. *Amer. J. Psychiat.*, 116: 641-644 (II A 3 g).

Lloyd, W. B., & Wise, H. B. (1968), The Montefiore experience. *Bull. N.Y. Acad. Med.*, 44:1353-1362 (II B 7).

Locke, B., Kramer, M., Timberlake, C., Pasamanick, B., & Smeltzer, D. (1958), Problems in interpretations of patterns of first admissions to Ohio state public mental hospitals for patients with schizophrenic reactions. *Psychiat. Res. Rep. No. 10.* Wash., D.C.: Amer. Psychiat. Assoc., pp. 172-196 (I A 1).

Loeb, M. B. (1956), Some dominant cultural themes in a psychiatric hospital. *Soc. Probs.*, 4:17-20 (I B 1).

———— (1957), Role definition in the social world of a psychiatric hospital. In: Greenblatt, M., Levinson, D. J., & Williams, R. H. (Eds.) (1957), pp. 14-19 (I B 1).

Lowenkopf, E. L., & Zwerling, I. (1971), Psychiatric services in a neighborhood health center. *Amer. J. Psychiat.*, 127:916-920 (II B 7).

Lubach, J. E., Bonn, E. M., Schiff, S. B., Larsen, E. E., & Braun, M. L. (1963), Action research improves nurse-resident relations. *Ment. Hosp.*, 14:627-631 (II C 2; I B 3; II A 3 g; II A 3 c).

Luezki, M. B. (1958), *Interdisciplinary Team Research: Methods and Problems.* N.Y.: N.Y. Univ. Press (II C 2; II A 2).

Luft, J. (1963), *Group Processes—An Introduction to Group Dynamics.* Palo Alto, Calif.: National Press (I B 3; II B 1; II C 1).

Lundstedt, S. (1965), Social psychological contributions to mental hospital administration. *Amer. J. Psychiat.*, 122:195-202 (I B 1; I B 2).

Lurie, A., Miller, J., Pinsky, L., Posner, W., & Vogelstein, H. (1956), The placement of discharged mental patients in foster homes: A cooperative project between mental hospital and family agency. *J. Hillside Hosp.*, 5:468 (II B 5; II B 6).

Macht, L. B. (1975), Beyond the mental health center: Planning for a community of neighborhoods. *Psychiat. Ann.*, 5:56-69 (I A 1; II B 7).

Macinnes, D., & Macaulay, K. (1963), Pattern for tomorrow. *Nurs. Times,* 59:868-870 (I A 1; I C 3).

Mackie, R. J. (1963), In Illinois: A fresh start in mental health. *Hospitals,* 37:45-58 (I A 1; I C 3).

MacKinnon, I. H. (1963), Progress report from Milledgeville State Hospital. *J. Med. Assoc. Ga.,* 52:868-870 (Cf., Medical Association of Georgia, 1959) (I A 1; I C 3).

Maddison, D. C. (1960), Blueprint for a model psychiatric hospital. *Med. J. Austral.,* 47:33-36 (I A 1; I C 3).

Mahrer, A. R. (1962), The psychodynamics of psychiatric hospital-ization. *J. Nerv. Ment. Dis.,* 135:354-360 (I C 3).

Main, T. F. (1946), The hospital as a therapeutic institution. *Bull. Menninger Clin.,* 10:66-70 (I C 3; II B 1; I B 1).

Maine, H. (1947), *If a Man Be Mad.* N.Y.: Doubleday (I A 1; I C 3).

Mako, A. E. (1961), Patient government: Development and out-growths. *Ment. Hosp.,* 12:30-32 (II B 3).

Malzberg, B. (1953), Rates of discharge and rates of mortality among first admissions to the New York civil state hospitals. *Ment. Hygiene,* 37:619-654 (I A 1).

Mandelbrote, B. (1958), An experiment in the rapid conversion of a closed mental hospital into an open-door hospital. *Ment. Hygiene,* 42:1 (II B 2).

———— (1959), Development of a comprehensive psychiatric com-munity service around the mental hospital. *Ment. Hygiene,* 43:368-377 (II B 6).

———— & Freeman, H. (1963), The closed group concept in open psychiatric hospitals. *Amer. J. Psychiat.,* 19:763-767 (II B 2; II B 1).

Mangum, M. M., Shrift, D., & Camp, W. P. (1963), "Out of the rut." *Ment. Hosp.,* 14:320-321 (I A 1; I C 3).

Mann, R. D. (1959), A review of the relationships between person-ality and performance in small groups. *Psychol. Bull.,* 56:241-270 (I B 3; II B 1).

Margolis, P. M., Daniels, R. M., Carson, R. C., & Meyer, G. G. (1963), The patient-staff meeting—a technique for encouraging communication in the psychiatric hospital. *Psychiatry,* 26:19-25 (II B 3; I B 3).

Marshall, J. A., & Schlesinger, H. J. (1949), Some implications of the concept of structure for the psychiatric team. Topeka: Winter VA Hospital (II A 2; I B 1; I B 3).

Martin, H. W. (1962), Structural sources of strain in a small psychi-atric hospital. *Psychiatry,* 25:3447-3453 (I B 1; I B 2; I B 3).

Martin, M. (1972), Community mental health centers: Coming to grips with big ideas. *Amer. J. Psychiat.,* 129:211-213 (II B 7).

Masserman, J. H. (1963), Psychiatric residency training for public institutional service. *Amer. J. Psychiat.,* 119:1038-1044 (II C 1).

Maxmen, J. S., Tucker, G. J., & LeBow, M. (1974), *Rational Hospi-tal Psychiatry,* N.Y.: Brunner/Mazel (I A 1).

May, P. R. A. (1963), Neurologic service develops in a state hospital. *Ment. Hosp.,* 14:644-646 (II A 3 d).

———— & Wilkinson, M. A. (1963), A new admission procedure. *Nurs. Outlook,* 11:355-358 (I C 3; I B 2).

McBee, M., & Frank, M. (1950), *Volunteer Participation in Psychiatric Hospital Services: Organization Manual and Program Guide.* N.Y.: Nat. Assoc. Ment. Health (II A 3 j).

McDermott, J. F., Jr., & Maretzki, T. W. (1975), Some guidelines for the training of foreign medical graduates: Results of a special project. *Amer. J. Psychiat.,* 132:658-661 (II C 1).

McGrabee, C. L. (1961), The ward community: A new route toward long-standing goals. *Ment. Hosp.,* 12:37-39 (II B 1).

McKerracher, D. G. (1949), A new program in the training and employment of ward personnel. *Amer. J. Psychiat.,* 106:259 (II A 3 h; I C 3).

―――― (1961), Psychiatric care in transition. *Ment. Hygiene,* 45:3-9 (I C 3).

McLary, R. (1961), Communication patterns as bases of systems of authority and power. In: Social Science Research Council Pamphlet No. 15. Quoted in Goffman, E. (1961), p. 286, fn. 147 (I B 1; I B 2).

McLaughlin, D. (1950), Contribution of the psychiatric nurse to the clinical team. In: *Education for Psychiatric Social Workers.* N.Y.: Amer. Assoc. Psychiat. Soc. Workers, pp. 54-58 (II A 3 g; II A 2).

McLean, R. (1958), Special areas involving mental hospital-community relationships. *Ment. Hosp.,* 9:54-60 (II B 6).

Mechanick, P., & Nathan, R. J. (1965), Is psychiatric hospitalization obsolete? *J. Nerv. Ment. Dis.,* 141:378-383 (I C 3; I A 1).

Medical Association of Georgia (1959), Report of M.A.G. Milledgeville Study Committee. (Recommendations for reorganization of Milledgeville State Hospital made by the State Medical Association.) *J. Med. Assoc. Ga.,* 48:275-285 (Cf. MacKinnon, I. H., 1963) (II B 6; I B 2; I A 1).

Menninger, K. (1949), The doctor as a leader. *Bull. Menninger Clin.,* 13:9-15 (I C 2).

Menninger, W. C. (1936), Psychiatric hospital treatment designed to meet unconscious needs. *Amer. J. Psychiat.,* 93:347-360 (I C 3; II B 1).

―――― (1939), Psychoanalytic principles in psychiatric hospital therapy. *Southern Med. J.,* 32:348-354 (II A 3 b; I C 3).

―――― (1942), The functions of the psychiatric hospital. *Bull. Menninger Clin.,* 6:109-116 (I C 3; I A 1).

Menninger, W. W. (1964), Staff expectations of a ward psychiatrist. *Ment. Hosp.,* 15:370-373 (I C 2; II A 3 c).

Mercier, C. A. (1894), *Lunatic Asylums: Organization and Management.* London: Charles Griffin (I B 2; I B 1; I A 1; I C 3).

Mereness, D. (1959), Factors influencing the nurse's role. *Ment. Hosp.,* 10:16-17 (II A 3 g).

Mering, O. von (1957), the social self-renewal of the mental patient and the volunteer movement. In: Greenblatt, M., Levinson, D. J., & Williams, R. H. (Eds.) (1957), pp. 585-593 (II A 3 j; I C 3; II B 6).

―――― & King, S. H. (1957a), A social classification of patients. In: *Remotivating the Mental Patient.* N.Y.: Russell Sage Found., pp. 27-47 (I B 1; I C 3).

―――― ―――― (1957b), The sick help the sicker. In: *Remotivating the Mental Patient.* N.Y.: Russell Sage Found., pp. 107-109 (II B 3).

Metcalf, G. R. (1961), The English open mental hospitals: Implications for American psychiatric services. *Milbank Memorial Fund Quart.,* 39:579-593 (II B 2).

Middleton, J. (1953), Prejudices and opinions of mental hospital employees regarding mental illness. *Amer. J. Psychiat.,* 110:133 (II A 3 m; I B 1).

Miles, M. B. (1959), *Learning to Work in Groups.* N.Y.: Columbia Univ. Press (I B 3; II B 1; II C 1).

―――― (1962), Human relations training: Current status. In: NTL Selected Reading Series, *Issues in Human Relations Training.* Vol. V. Wash., D.C.: Nat. Training Labs.-Nat. Educ. Assoc., pp. 3-13 (I B 3; II B 1; II C 1).

Miller, A. A. (1964), Therapeutic resources in state hospitals: The psychiatric nurse. *Compr. Psychiat.,* 5:122-127 (II A 3 g).

―――― & Sabshin, M. (1963), Psychotherapy in psychiatric hospitals. A proposed model for psychiatrist-nurse-patient interaction. *Arch. Gen. Psychiat.,* 9:53-63 (II A 2; II A 3 g).

Milnar, G., Kumar, K., & Bakker, A. H. (1963), The team system and admissions to a mental hospital. *Brit. Med. J.,* 5327:389-390 (II A 1).

Mishler, E. G. (1955), The nursing service and the aims of a psychiatric hospital: Orientations of ward personnel and the care and rehabilitation of psychiatric patients. *Amer. J. Psychiat.,* 111:664 (II A 3 g; II A 3 i; II C 1; I C 3).

―――― & Trapp (1956), Status and inter-relation in a psychiatric hospital. *Human Relations,* 9:187-205 (I B 1).

―――― & Waxler, E. G. (1963), Decision processes in psychiatric hospitalizations: Patients referred, accepted, and admitted to a psychiatric hospital. *Amer. Sociol. Rev.,* 78:576-587 (I A 1).

Modlin, H. C. (1951), Integration of educational and administrative psychiatry. *Psychiat. Quart.,* 25:475-483 (II C 1; I B 2; I B 3).

———— & Faris, M. (1954), Follow-up study of a psychiatric team. *Bull. Menninger Clin.*, 18:242-251 (II A 2).

———— ———— (1956), Group adaptation and integration in psychiatric team practice. *Psychiatry*, 19:97-103 (II A 2; I B 3).

————, Gardner, R., & Faris, M. (1958), Implications of a therapeutic process in evaluations by psychiatric teams. *Amer. J. Orthopsychiat.*, 28:647-655 (II A 2; I C 3).

Montonaro, M. O. (1964), High school students as ancillary staff in a psychiatric hospital. Presented to the Annual Meeting of the American Psychiatric Association, Los Angeles, May 8 (II A 2; I C 3; II A 3 j).

Moore, R. A. (1964), State hospitals and alcoholism — a nation-wide survey of treatment techniques and results. Presented to the Annual Meeting of the American Psychiatric Association, Los Angeles, May 4 (I C 3).

Moran, M. J., & Leopold, W. D. (1963), An educational workshop for relatives. *Ment. Hosp.*, 14:280-282 (II B 4; II C 1).

Morgan, N. C., & Johnson, N. A. (1957), Failures in psychiatry: The chronic patient. *Amer. J. Psychiat.*, 113:824-830 (I C 3).

Morgan, R. D., & Cook, L. R. (1963), Relationship of methods of admission to length of stay in state hospitals. *Public Health Rep.*, 78:619-629 (I A 1; I C 3).

Morgan, T. M., & Hall, B. H. (1950), Report of an experiment in psychiatric aide training. *Bull. Menninger Clin.*, 14:27-33 (II A 3 i; II C 1).

Morimoto, F. R. (1955), A technique for measuring interactions of patients and personnel in mental hospitals. *Nurs. Res.*, 4:74-78 (II C 2; I B 1).

Moss, G. R., & Boren, J. J. (1971), Specifying critieria for completion of psychiatric treatment. *Arch. Gen. Psychiat.*, 24:441-447 (I C 3).

Mounts, A. (1961), The librarian in the psychiatric hospital. *Hosp. Progr.*, 42:106-108 (II A 3 j).

Muller, T. (1950), *Mental Institutions: Historical Background — Nature and Direction of Psychiatric Nursing*. Philadelphia: Lippincott (II A 3 g; I A 1).

Mumford, E., Brown, F., & Kaufman, M. R. (1971), A hospital-based mental health project. *Amer. J. Psychiat.*, 127:920-924 (II B 6; II B 7).

Murphy, B. W. (1951), Some interpersonal processes and situations delaying discharge from a psychiatric institute. *Dis. Nerv. Syst.*, 12:273 (I B 1; I A 1).

Murphy, G. E., & Hunt, R. G. (1964), Milieu therapy: Theoretical and practical considerations in its application. In: Wessen, A. F. (1964), pp. 176-184 (II B 1).

Murray, E., & Cohen, M. (1959), Mental illness, milieu therapy and social organization in ward groups. *J. Abn. Psychol.,* 58:48 (II B 1; I B 1).

Myers, J. M. (1951), Coordination of occupational therapy with the nursing and medical staffs in a teaching psychiatric hospital. *Occup. Ther. Rehab.,* 30:224-229 (II A 2; I B 3; II A 3 h; II A 3 g; II A 3 c).

―――― & Smith, L. H. (1959), Administrative psychiatry. *Amer. J. Psychiat.,* 115:647-649 (I B 2).

―――― ―――― (1961), Administrative psychiatry. *Amer. J. Psychiat.,* 117:649-651 (I B 2).

―――― ―――― (1963), Administrative psychiatry. *Amer. J. Psychiat.,* 119:675-677 (I B 2).

Naboisek, H., Simmons, O. G., Mathews, D. M., & Cath, S. H. (1957), Hospital and post-hospital experience. In: Greenblatt, M., Levinson, D. J., & Williams, R. H. (Eds.) (1957), pp. 565-576 (II B 5; II B 6).

Nadel, S. F. (1953), Social control and self-regulation. *Soc. Forces,* 31:265-273 (II B 3).

Nakagama, H., & Hudziak, B. (1963), Effect of increases in numbers of nursing personnel on utilization of time in a psychiatric unit. *Nurs. Res.,* 12:106-108 (II A 3 g; I C 3; II A 1).

National Association for Mental Health (1946 & 1950), *Handbook for Psychiatric Aides.* Section one: A general guide to work in mental hospitals, 1946. Section two: Care of the overactive and disturbed patient, 1950. N.Y.: Nat. Assoc. Ment. Health (II A 3 i; I C 3).

―――― (1952), *Twelve Facts about Mental Illness.* N.Y.: Nat. Assoc. Ment. Health (I C 3; II B 6).

―――― (1960), *Recruitment and Retention of Volunteers for Service in Veterans Administration Hospitals, 1960.* N.Y.: Nat. Assoc. Ment. Health (II A 3 j; I C 1).

―――― (1961), *Volunteer Services in Mental Hospitals.* N.Y.: Nat. Assoc. Ment. Health (II A 3 j).

―――― (1963), The unit plan. Conference transcript of the Mental Health Association of Southeastern Pennsylvania. N.Y.: Nat. Assoc. Ment. Health (II A 1).

National Institute of Mental Health (1964), Regulations for community mental health centers act of 1963, Title II. *Federal Register,* May 6, pp. 5951-5956 (II B 7).

_____ (1969), *Length of Stay for Discharges from General Hospital Psychiatric Inpatient Units, United States, 1970-71.* Statistical Note 70. Wash., D.C.: U.S. Govt. Printing Office (I A 1).

_____ (1972), *Staffing Patterns in Mental Health Facilities.* Wash., D.C.: NIMH, Series B, No. 6 (I A 1; I C 1).

_____ (1974), *Inventory for Mental Health Facilities.* Wash., D.C.: NIMH, Biometry Branch (I A 1).

Newcomb, E. P. (1961), Personalization of patient care in a mental hospital. *Ment. Hosp.,* 12:37-38 (I C 3; I A 1; I C 1).

Newton, H. J. (1967), The comprehensive mental health center: Uncharted horizons for inpatient services. *Amer. J. Psychiat.,* 123:1210-1219 (II B 6; II B 7).

Noroian, E. H. (1962), Research. In: Owen, J. K. (Ed.), *Modern Concepts of Hospital Administration.* Philadelphia: Saunders, p. 736 (II C 2; I B 2).

Novey, R. (1960), In-patient psychiatric care in a state hospital. *Maryland Med. J.,* 9:441-446 (I C 3).

Nurnberger, J. I., Zuckerman, M., Norton, J. A., & Brittain, H. M. (1961), Certain sociocultural and economic factors influencing utilization of state institutional facilities in Indiana. *Amer. J. Psychiat.,* 117:1065-1074 (I A 1; II B 6).

O'Dea, J. F. (1961), Reducing overcrowding in Clonmel Mental Hospital. *J. Irish Med. Assoc.,* 48:132-136 (I A 1).

Odegard, O. (1968), The pattern of discharge and readmission in Norwegian Hospitals, 1936-1963. *Amer. J. Psychiat.,* 125:333-340 (I A 1).

Odenheimer, J. F. (1965), Day hospital as an alternative to the psychiatric ward. *Arch. Gen. Psychiat.,* 13:46-53 (II B 5).

O'Neill, F. J. (1960), The mental hospital: Cornerstone for community services. *Amer. J. Psychiat.,* 116:810-813 (II B 6).

Opler, M. K. (1956), *Culture, Psychiatry, and Human Values.* Springfield, Ill.: Charles C Thomas (II B 6; I B 1; I C 3).

Ortega, M. J. (1962), Open-ward management of disturbed mental patients of both sexes. *Ment. Hygiene,* 46:48-58 (II B 2; I C 3).

Osmond, H. (1957), Function as the basis of psychiatric ward design. *Ment. Hosp.,* 41:23-30 (I C 3; II B 1).

Overholser, W. (1939), The desiderata of central administrative control of state mental hospitals. *Amer. J. Psychiat.,* 96:517-534 (I B 2).

_____ (1942), The function of the state hospital as an educational and social agency. *JAMA,* 118:1027-1033 (II C 1; II B 6).

_____ (1953), Administrative psychiatry. In: Whitehorn, J. C., Braceland, F. J., Lippard, V. W., & Malamud, W. (Eds.) (1953), pp. 114-116 (I B 2).

_____ (1961), The changing scene: The volunteer as an index. *Ment. Hosp.*, 12:26-28 (II A 3 j).

Owen, J. K. (Ed.) (1962), *Modern Concepts of Hospital Administration*. Philadelphia: Saunders (I B 2).

Ozarin, L. D., & Brown, B. S. (1965), New directions in community mental health programs. *Amer. J. Orthopsychiat.*, 35: 10-17 (II B 7).

_____ , Feldman, S., & Spaner, F. E. (1971), Experience with community mental health centers. *Amer. J. Psychiat.*, 127:912-916 (II B 7).

_____ & Levenson, A. I. (1969), The future of the public mental hospital. *Amer. J. Psychiat.*, 125:1647-1652 (I A 1).

_____ & Taube, C. (1974), Psychiatric inpatients: Who, where and future. *Amer. J. Psychiat.*, 131:98-104 (I A 1).

Padula, H. (1960), Problems in the team treatment of adults in state mental hospitals. Panel, 1958. 5. Comments on the state hospital team by a social worker. *Amer. J. Orthopsychiat.*, 30:109-112 (II A 2; I B 3; I C 3).

Panel discussion (1959), The psychiatric ward administrator. *Ment. Hosp.*, 10(4):20-23 (II A 3 c; I C 2).

_____ (1963), Milieu therapy—a dialogue. *Ment. Hosp.*, 14:337-354 (II B 1).

Parker, S. (1959), The natural history of a disorganization on a psychiatric ward. *Psychiatry*, 22:65-79 (I B 1).

Parkes, C. M. (1963), Interhospital and intrahospital variations in the diagnosis and severity of schizophrenia. *Brit. J. Prev. Soc. Med.*, 17:85-89 (I A 1).

Parloff, M. B. (1960), The impact of ward-milieu philosophies on nursing-role concepts. *Psychiatry*, 23:141-151 (II B 1; II A 3 g).

Parsons, T. (1952), The superego and the theory of social systems. *Psychiatry*, 15:15-25 (I B 1; II B 6).

_____ (1957), The mental hospital as a type of organization. In: Greenblatt, M., Levinson, D. J., & Williams, R. H. (Eds.) (1957), pp. 108-129 (I B 1).

Pasamanick, B. (Ed.) (1959), *Epidemiology of Mental Disorder*. Wash., D.C.: Amer. Assoc. Adv. Sci. (I A 1).

_____ , Scarpitti, F. R., & Dinitz, S. (1967), *Schizophrenics in the Community: An Experimental Study in the Prevention of Hospitalization*. N.Y.: Appleton-Century-Crofts (II B 7).

Pascoe, H. (1963), Group "therapy" with student nurses. *Canad. Psychiat. Assoc. J.*, 8:205-210 (II A 3 g; II C 1).

Pearl, A., & Riessman, F. (1966), *New Careers for the Poor: The Non-Professional in Human Service.* N.Y.: Free Press (II A 3 i).

Peck, H., Roman, M., & Kaplan, S. R. (1967), Community action programs and the comprehensive mental health center. In: Greenblatt, M., Emory, P. E., & Glueck, B. C. (Eds.), Poverty and mental health. *Res. Rep. Amer. Psychiat. Assoc.*, 21:103-121 (II B 7).

Peplau, H. E. (1956), Present-day trends in psychiatric nursing. *Neuropsychiat.*, 3:190-204 (II A 3 g).

———— (1960), Problems in the team treatment of adults in state mental hospitals. Panel, 1958. 4. Must laboring together be called "teamwork?" *Amer. J. Orthopsychiat.*, 30:103-108 (II A 2; I B 3; I C 3).

Pepper, B. W. (1975), The effect of the right to treatment on psychiatry. Presented to the Annual Meeting of the American Psychiatric Association, Anaheim, Calif., May 5-9. *Scientific Proceedings in Summary Form.* Wash., D.C.: Amer. Psychiat. Assoc., pp. 175-176 (I C 3).

Perkins, C. T. (1950), Why state hospital superintendents fail. *Amer. J. Psychiat.*, 107:170 (I B 2).

Perkins, G. L. (1952), A plan for training in dynamic psychiatry for state hospitals. *Ill. Med. J.*, 101:261 (II C 3; II C 1).

Perkins, M. (1959), Volunteer workers in mental hospitals. *Nurs. Outlook*, 7:288-290 (II A 3 j).

Perlin, S. (1960), Perception and tolerance of psychopathology by a heterogeneous group on a hospital ward. *Psychiatry*, 23:225-227 (I B 1).

Perretz, E. A. (1960), Care of the mentally ill in Ontario: The volunteer in psychiatric service. *Canad. Hosp.*, 37:51-52 (II A 3 j; I C 3).

Perry, S. E., & Shea, G. N. (1957), Social controls and psychiatric theory in a ward setting. *Psychiatry*, 20:221-247 (I B 1; II B 1; II B 3).

Person, P. (1962), Geographic variation in first admission rates to a state mental hospital. *Public Health Rep.*, 77:719-731. Wash., D.C.: U.S. Public Health Serv. (I A 1).

Peterson, C. L. (1963), Defining the ideal psychiatric team. *Provo Papers* (Utah State Hospital), 7:70-77 (II A 2).

Pfeffer, P. A., Margolin, B. A., Stotsky, B. A., & Mason, A. S.

(Eds.)(1957), *Member-Employee Program: A New Approach to the Rehabilitation of the Chronic Mental Patient.* Brockton, Mass.: VA Hospital (II B 3; II A 3 h).

Phillips, F., & May, S. B. (1957), A study of the transfer of long-hospitalized patients to a convalescent service. *Amer. J. Psychiat.,* 114:344-350 (II B 5).

Phillips, J. (1961), *Ten Years with Trained Volunteers.* Chicago: Dept. Ment. Health (II A 3 j).

Pinderhughes, C. A., Goodglass, H., Mayo, C., Greenberg, R. M., & Friedman, H. L. (1966), A study of childhood origins of patients' ward relationships. *J. Nerv. Ment. Dis.,* 142:140-147 (II B 3).

Pine, F. (1955), Conceptions of the mentally ill and the self: A study of psychiatric aides. Cambridge, Mass.: Unpublished doctoral dissertation, Harvard Univ. (II A 3 i; I B 1).

———— & Levinson, D. J. (1957), Two patterns of ideology, role conception, and personality among mental hospital aides. In: Greenblatt, M., Levinson, D. J., & Williams, R. H. (Eds.) (1957), pp. 208-217 (II A 3 i; I B 1).

Pinsker, H., Robbins, E., & Kleinerman, G. (1972), Psychiatric hospitalization: Role of administration policy. *N.Y. State J. Med.,* 72:1764-1768 (I B 1; I B 2).

Pishkin, V., & Dredge, T. T. (1963), Temporal and demographic correlates of critical incidents with neuropsychiatric patients. *J. Clin. Psychol.,* 19:230-235 (I B 1).

————, Olson, L. O., & Jacobs, D. F. (1961), An objective attempt to analyze emotional interactions between psychiatric patients and nursing staff. *J. Clin. Psychol.,* 17:383-388 (II A 3 g).

Pitt, B., & Markowe, M. (1963), A new pattern in day hospital development. The West Middlesex Day Hospital. *Brit. J. Psychiat.,* 109:29-36 (II B 5).

Polansky, N. A., Lippitt, R., & Redl, F. (1950), An investigation of behavioral contagion in groups. *Human Relations,* 3:319-348 (Cf. also Stanton, A. H., & Schwartz, M. S. [1954], pp. 395ff.) (I B 1).

————, White, R. S., & Miller, S. C. (1957), Determinants of the role-image of the patient in a psychiatric hospital. In: Greenblatt, M., Levinson, D. J., & Williams, R. H. (Eds.) (1957), pp. 380-401 (I B 1).

Pollock, H. M. (Ed.) (1936), *Family Care of Mental Patients.* Utica, N.Y.: State Hosp. Press (II B 5; II B 4).

Pratt, S., & Delange, W. (1963), The admission-therapy group. Treatment of choice at a state hospital. *Ment. Hosp.,* 14:222-224 (I C 3).

———, Scott, G., Treesh, E., Khanna, J., Lesher, T., Khanna, P., Gardiner, G., & Wright, W. (1960), The mental hospital and the "treatment-field." *J. Psychol. Studies,* 11: Suppl. No. 8 (I B 1; I C 3; II B 1).

Preston, G. H. (1948), Integrating factors in psychiatric procedures. *Ment. Hygiene,* 32:407-410 (I B 3; I C 3; II B 1).

Prince, R. M., Ackerman, R. E., & Barksdale, B. S. (1973), Collaborative provision of aftercare services. *Amer. J. Psychiat.,* 130:930-932 (II B 5; II B 6).

Public Health Service (1947), *Patients in Mental Institutions.* Wash., D.C.: Federal Security Agency (I A 1).

——— (1953), *Proceedings of the Second Conference of Mental Hospital Administrators and Statisticians.* Wash., D.C.: Federal Security Agency (I A 1; I B 2).

Pugh, T. F., & McMahon, B. (1962), *Epidemiological Findings in United States Mental Hospital Data.* Boston: Little, Brown (I A 1).

——— ——— (1967), Measurement of discontinuity of psychiatric inpatient care. *Public Health Rep.,* 82:533-538 (I C 3).

Pumpian-Mindlin, E. (1964), Resident education in social and community psychiatry — problems of professional identity. Presented to the Annual Meeting of the American Psychiatric Association, Los Angeles, May 7 (II C 1; II B 7).

Puthu, B. (1959), The state mental hospital. *Burma Med. J.,* 7:199-201 (I A 1; I C 3).

Rabiner, E. L., Gomaz, E., & Gralnick, A. (1964), The therapeutic community as an insight catalyst — expanding the transferential field. *Amer. J. Psychother.,* 18:244-258 (II B 1).

———, Molinski, H., & Gralnick, A. (1962), Conjoint family therapy in the inpatient setting. *Amer. J. Psychother.,* 18:244 (II B 4).

Rada, R. T. (1975), Preliminary report of the task force on right to treatment. Presented to the Annual Meeting of the American Psychiatric Association, Anaheim, Calif., May 5-9. *Scientific Proceedings in Summary Form.* Wash., D.C.: Amer. Psychiat. Assoc., pp. 174-175 (I C 3).

Rapoport, R. N. (1963), Principles for developing a therapeutic community. In: Masserman, J. H. (Ed.), *Current Psychiatric Therapies,* 3:244-256. N.Y.: Grune & Stratton (II B 1).

_____ & Rapoport, R. S. (1957), "Democratization" and authority in a therapeutic community. *Behav. Sci.,* 2:128-133 (II B 1).

_____ & Skellern, E. (1957), Some therapeutic functions of administrative disturbance. *Admin. Sci. Quart.,* 2:84-85 (I B 2; I C 3; I B 1).

Raskin, N. (1958), Non-restraint. *Amer. J. Psychiat.,* 115:471 (II B 2; I C 3; II B 2).

Ratcliff, R. A. W. (1962), The open door—ten years' experience in Dingleton. *Lancet,* 2:188-190 (II B 2).

Ray, E. (1962), The autonomous unit system at the Ontario Hospital, New Toronto: I. *Canad. Psychiat. Assoc. J.,* 7:56-66 (II A 1).

Ray, I. (1873), Ideal character of the officers of a hospital for the insane. *Amer. J. Insanity,* 30:67 (I B 2; I C 2).

Redl, F. (1942), Group emotion and leadership. *Psychiatry,* 5:573-596 (I B 3; I C 2; I B 2).

Redlich, F. C. (Ed.) (1969), *Social Psychiatry.* Assoc. Research Nerv. Ment. Dis., Res. Public. Series, vol. 47. Baltimore: Williams & Wilkins (II B 1).

_____ & Astrachan, B. (1969), Group dynamics training. *Amer. J. Psychiat.,* 125:1501-1507 (II B 1; II C 1).

_____ & Pepper, M. (1968), Are social psychiatry and community psychiatry subspecialties of psychiatry? *Amer. J. Psychiat.,* 124: 1343-1350 (II B 7).

Rees, T. P. (1957), Some observations on the psychiatric patient, the mental hospital, and the community. In: Greenblatt, M., Levinson, D. J., & Williams, R. H. (Eds.) (1957), pp. 527-529 (I B 1; II B 6).

_____ & Glatt, M. M. (1955), The organization of a mental hospital on the basis of group participation. *Internat. J. Group Psychother.,* 5:157 (I B 1; I B 3; II B 1).

_____ _____ (1956), Mental hospitals. In: Slavson, S. R. (Ed.), *Fields of Group Psychotherapy.* N.Y.: Internat. Univ. Press, Chap. 2 (I A 1; I C 3).

Reich, R. (1973), Care of the chronically mentally ill—a national disgrace. *Amer. J. Psychiat.,* 130:911-912 (I A 1).

Reidy, J. P. (1964), *Zone Mental Health Centers—The Illinois Concept.* Springfield, Ill.: Charles C Thomas (II B 7).

Reinert, R. E., Vernallis, F. F., & Marler, D. C. (1964), The weekend hospital. Presented to the Annual Meeting of the American Psychiatric Association, Los Angeles, May 8 (II B 5).

Reinherz, H. (1962), Leadership of student volunteers. *Ment. Hosp.*, 13:600-602 (II A 3 j; I C 2).

Reisman, D. (1959), Some observations on interviewing in a state mental hospital. *Bull. Menninger Clin.*, 23:7-19 (I C 3).

Remington, F. B. (1963), "Walkouts" and the open hospital: A three month survey. *Psychiat. Quart.*, 37:128-133 (II B 2).

Render, H. W. (1947), *Nurse-Patient Relationships in Psychiatry.* N.Y.: McGraw-Hill (II A 3 g).

Rennie, T. A. C. (1955), Social psychiatry, a definition. *Internat. J. Soc. Psychiat.*, 1:5-13 (II B 1).

Retznikoff, M., Brady, J. P., & Zeller, W. W. (1959a), The psychiatric attitudes battery: A procedure for assessing attitudes toward psychiatric treatment and hospitals. *J. Clin. Psychol.*, 15:260-266 (II C 2; I B 1; I C 3).

———— ———— ———— (1959b), Attitudinal factors influencing outcome of treatment of hospitalized psychiatric patients. *J. Clin. Exper. Psychopath.*, 20:326-334 (I C 3).

Reuther, W. P. (1969), The health care crisis: Where do we go from here? *Amer. J. Public Health,* 59:12-20 (II B 7).

Rice, C. E., Klett, S. L., Berger, D. G., Sewall, L. G., & Lemkau, P. V. (1963), The Ward Evaluation Scale. *J. Clin. Psychol.*, 19:251-258 (I B 1; I C 3).

Richardson, H. B. (1945), *Patients Have Families.* N.Y.: Commonwealth Fund (II B 4).

Richman, A., & Pinsker, H. (1973), Utilization review of psychiatric inpatient care. *Amer. J. Psychiat.*, 130:900-903 (I C 3).

Rickman, J. (1950), The factor of number in individual and group dynamics. *J. Ment. Sci.*, 96:770-773 (I B 3; I A 1).

Riessman, C. K. (1970), The supply-demand dilemma in community mental health centers. *Amer. J. Orthopsychiat.*, 40:858-869 (II B 7).

Riessman, F., Cohen, J., & Pearl, A. (Eds.) (1964), *Mental Health of the Poor.* N.Y.: Free Press (II B 7).

———— & Hallowitz, E. (1967), The neighborhood service center: An innovation in preventive psychiatry. *Amer. J. Psychiat.*, 123:1408-1413 (II B 7).

Rinsley, D. B. (1963), Psychiatric hospital treatment. *Arch. Gen. Psychiat.*, 9:489-496 (I C 3).

Rioch, D. McK., & Stanton, A. H. (1953), Milieu therapy. *Psychiatry,* 16:65-72 (II B 1).

Robbins, C. A. (1963), A therapeutic milieu in a continued treatment service. *Ment. Hosp.*, 14:494-495 (II B 1; I C 3).

Robbins, L. (1963), The contributions of psychoanalysis in psychiatric hospital treatment. *J. Hillside Hosp.*, 12: Nos. 3 & 4 (II A 3 b; I C 3).

Roberts, E. L., & Lindsay, J. S. (1962), The mental hospital: Structure, function, and communication. *Brit. J. Med. Psychol.*, 35:155-164 (I B 1; I B 3).

Robinson, A., Mellow, J., Hurteau, P., & Fried, M. (1955), Research in psychiatric nursing. *Amer. J. Nursing*, 55:441-444, 572-575, 704-707 (II C 2; II A 3 g).

Robinson, A. M. (1954), *The Psychiatric Aide—A Textbook of Patient Care.* Philadelphia: Lippincott (II A 3 i; I C 3).

Robinson, R. L., Branson, R., Chalmers, R., Greenberg, P. M., & Mackin, M. C. (1963), The public image of institutions. *Ment. Hosp.*, 14:125-126 (I A 1).

Rockefeller, Mrs. W. (1958), *New Roles for Trained Volunteer Workers in Mental Health.* Austin, Tex.: Hogg Found. Mental Health, Univ. of Texas (II A 3 j; I C 3).

Rogers, F. R. (1963), Patients respond to music program. *Ment. Hosp.*, 14:642-644 (II A 3 h).

Rome, H. P. (1965), Problems in the establishment of community mental health centers. *Southern Med. J.*, 58:985-991 (II B 7).

Ropschitz, D. H. (1963), On reducing the mental hospital population in Great Britain. *Internat. J. Soc. Psychiat.*, 9:58-63 (I A 1).

Rose, A. (Ed.) (1955), *Mental Health and Mental Disorder.* N.Y.: Norton (I A 1; I C 3).

Rosenbaum, M., & Zwerling, I. (1964), Impact of social psychiatry: Effect on a psychoanalytically-oriented department of psychiatry. *Arch. Gen. Psychiat.*, 11:31-39 (II A 3 b; II B 1).

Rosenberg, B. G., Balogh, J. K., Gerjuoy, H., Bond, J., & McDevitt, R. (1962), The DL scale: The measurement of clinical status of a psychiatric ward. *J. Clin. Psychol.*, 18:290-294 (II C 2).

Rosengren, W. R. (1961), Status stress and role contradictions: Emergent professionalization in psychiatric hospitals. *Ment. Hygiene*, 45:28-39 (I B 1; I C 2).

Ross, M. (1963), Some correctible images of psychiatric patients, physicians and hospitals. *Amer. J. Psychiat.*, 119:954-959 (II B 6).

Rothaus, P., Morton, R. B., Johnson, D. L., Cleveland, S. E., & Lyle, F. A. (1963), Human relations training for psychiatric patients. *Arch. Gen. Psychiat.*, 8:572-581 (I B 3; II C 1).

Rothstein, C. (1962), A psychiatric continued treatment ward program. *Psychiat. Quart.*, 36:703 (I C 3).

_____ (1966), Four-year follow-up of a non-traditional treatment program for chronic psychiatric patients. *J. Nerv. Ment. Dis.*, 142:355-368 (I C 3; II B 5).

Rowell, J. T. (1955), An approach to the treatment of massive mental hospital population. *Ment. Hygiene*, 39:622-630 (I A 1; I C 3).

Rowland, H. (1938), Interaction processes in a state mental hospital. *Psychiatry*, 1:323-337 (I B 1).

_____ (1939a), Friendship patterns in a state mental hospital. *Psychiatry*, 2:326-373 (II B 3; I B 1).

_____ (1939b), Segregated communities and mental health. In: Moulton, F. R. (ed.), *Mental Health Publications of the American Association for the Advancement of Science*, No. 9. N.Y.: Amer. Assoc. Adv. Sci. (II B 6; I A 2).

Rubenstein, R., & Lasswell, H. (1966), *The Sharing of Power in a Psychiatric Hospital*. New Haven: Yale Univ. Press (I B 2; II A 1).

Rubin, B., & Goldberg, A. (1963), An investigation of openness in the psychiatric hospital. *Arch. Gen. Psychiat.*, 8:269-276 (II B 2).

Rudquist, B. J. (1962), Preparing volunteers for psychiatric service. *Auxiliary Leader*, Jan. (II A 3 j).

Rudy, L. H., & Smith, J. A. (1961), Modern concepts of hospital therapy. *Curr. Psychiat. Ther.*, 1:190-195 (I C 3).

Ruesch, J. (1956), Creation of a multidisciplinary team. *Psychosom. Med.*, 18:105-112 (II A 2).

_____ (1965), Social psychiatry—an overview. *Arch. Gen. Psychiat.*, 12:501-509 (II B 1).

_____ (1966), Hospitalization and social disability. *J. Nerv. Ment. Dis.*, 142:203-214 (II B 1).

_____ & Bareson, G. (1949), Structure and process in social relations. *Psychiatry*, 12:105-124 (I B 1; II B 1).

Rushing, W. A. (1964), *The Psychiatric Professions: Power, Conflict, and Adaptation in a Psychiatric Hospital Staff*. Chapel Hill, N. C.: Univ. North Carolina Press (I B 1; I B 3; I B 2).

Russell, W. L. (1949), The role of medical administration in psychiatric hospital treatment. *Amer. J. Psychiat.*, 105:721 (I B 2; I C 3; I C 2).

Rutman, I. D., & Egan, K. L. (1975; The future role of state mental hospitals: A national survey of planning and program trends. Philadelphia: Horizon House Inst. Res. & Devel. (Reviewed in *Psychiat. News*, 10:1 & 16, Dec. 3.) (I A 1).

Ryan, J. H. (1962), The therapeutic value of the closed ward. *J. Nerv. Ment. Dis.*, 134:263-267 (II B 2).

———— (1964), Educational television in psychiatry. Presented to the Annual Meeting of the American Psychiatric Association, Los Angeles, May 5 (II C 1).

Ryan, W. (1969), Community care in historical perspective. *Canad. Ment. Health,* 17: Suppl. 60 (II B 7).

Ryniker, R. (1962), The management analyst: A new member of the hospital team. *Ment. Hosp.,* 13:254-255 (I B 2; II A 2; II A 3 b).

Sabagh, G., Dingman, H. F., & Windle, C. D. (1963), Variations in the image of a mental hospital and situational bias. *Ment. Hygiene,* 47:96-102 (I B 1).

Sabshin, M. (1962), Research projects in private hospitals and psychiatric units. *Hosp. Progr.,* 43:110-115 (II C 2).

———— (1969), The anti-community health "movement." *Amer. J. Psychiat.,* 125:1005-1012 (II B 7).

Sadoff, R. L. (1975), The right to treatment: What it is and what it is not. Presented to the Annual Meeting of the American Psychiatric Association, Anaheim, Calif., May 5-9. *Scientific Proceedings in Summary Form.* Wash., D.C.: Amer. Psychiat. Assoc., pp. 172-173 (I C 3).

Sainsbury, P. (1969), Social and community psychiatry. *Amer. J. Psychiat.,* 125:1226-1231 (II B 7).

Sampson, H., Ross, D., Engle, B., et al. (1957), *A Study of Suitability for Outpatient Clinic Treatment of State Mental Hospital Admissions.* Res. Rep. No. 1. Sacramento: State of Calif. Dept. Ment. Hygiene (II B 5).

Sandall, H., et al. (1975), The St. Louis community homes program: Graduated support for long-term care. *Amer. J. Psychiat.,* 132: 617-622 (II B 5).

Saucier, D. S., & Hoda, C. P. (1960), Patients help patients. *Ment. Hosp.,* 11:19-21 (II B 3).

Schacht, L., & Blacker, M. (1969), Leadership effect on the staff conference process. *Arch. Gen. Psychiat.,* 20:358-364 (I C 2).

Schaffer, L., & Myers, J. K. (1954), Psychotherapy and social satisfaction: An empirical study of practice in a psychiatric outpatient clinic. *Psychiatry,* 17:83-93 (II B 7).

Scher, M., & Johnson, M. H. (1963), Divergent staff attitudes spark a ward revolt. *Ment. Hosp.,* 14:492-494 (I B 1).

Scherl, D. J. (1966), Mental health implications of the Economic Opportunity Act. In: Lubin, B. (Ed.), *Proceedings of Conference of Psychology Program Directors and Consultants in State, Federal, and Territorial Mental Health Programs.* Indianapolis: Ind. Dept. Ment. Health (II B 7).

_____ & English, J. T. (1969), Community mental health and comprehensive health service programs for the poor. *Amer. J. Psychiat.*, 125:1666-1674 (II B 7).

Schiff, S. B. (1969), A therapeutic community in an open state hospital—administrative framework for social psychiatry. *Hosp. & Commun. Psychiat.*, 20 (II B 1; II B 2).

Schmitt, M. S., & Gordon, J. B. (1958), A cooperative plan for bettering care to the mentally ill. *Nurs. Outlook*, 6:521-522 (II A 3 g; I C 3).

Schneider, I. (1963), The use of patients to act out professional conflicts. *Psychiatry*, 26:88-94 (I B 1).

Schoenberg, B., Pettit, H. F., & Carr, A. C. (1968), *Teaching Psychosocial Aspects of Patient Care.* N.Y.: Columbia Univ. Press (I C 3; II B 1).

Schreier, A. J., & Lozito, D. (1963), Integrating clinical research with treatment. *Ment. Hosp.*, 14:573-577 (II C 2; I C 3).

Schulberg, H. C., & Baker, F. (1975), *The Mental Hospital and Human Services.* N.Y.: Behav. Publ. (I A 1).

_____ , Notman, R., & Bookin, E. (1967), Treatment services at a mental hospital in transition. *Amer. J. Psychiat.*, 124:506-513 (I C 3).

Schwartz, A., & Swartzburg, M. (1975), A five-year study of brief hospitalization. Presented to the Annual Meeting of the American Psychiatric Association, Anaheim, Calif., May 5-9. *Scientific Proceedings in Summary Form.* Wash., D.C.: Amer. Psychiat. Assoc., pp. 220-221 (I C 3).

Schwartz, C. G. (1953), *Rehabilitation of Mental Hospital Patients.* Wash., D.C.: Public Health Monogr. No. 17, Public Health Serv., Dept. HEW, U.S. Govt. Printing Office (I C 3; II B 1; I B 1).

_____ (1956), The stigma of mental illness. *J. Rehab.*, 22:7-8, 20-22, 28-29 (II B 6).

_____ (1957), Problems for psychiatric nurses in playing a new role on a mental hospital ward. In: Greenblatt, M., Levinson, D. J., & Williams, R. H. (Eds.) (1957), pp. 402-426 (II A 3 g; I C 3).

_____ , Schwartz, M. S., & Stanton, A. H. (1951), A study of need-fulfillment on a mental hospital ward. *Psychiatry*, 14:223-242 (I B 1; I C 3; II B 1).

Schwartz, D. A., & Waldron, R. (1963), Overprotection in the psychiatric hospital. *Psychiat. Quart.*, 37:282-296 (I C 3).

Schwartz, M. S. (1957a), Patient demands in a mental hospital context. *Psychiatry,* 20:249-261 (I C 3; I B 1).

―――― (1957b), What is a therapeutic milieu? In: Greenblatt, M., Levinson, D. J., & Williams, R. H. (Eds.) (1957), pp. 130-144 (II B 1).

―――― (1960), Problems in the team treatment of adults in state mental hospitals. I. Functions of the team in the state mental hospital. *Amer. J. Orthopsychiat.,* 30:100-102 (II A 2; I B 3; I C 3).

―――― & Schwartz, C. G. (1959), Considerations in determining a model for the mental hospital. *Amer. J. Psychiat.,* 116:435-437 (Cf. Schwartz, M. S., & Schwartz, C. G., 1960) (I B 1; I C 3; I A 1).

―――― ―――― (1960), *Considerations in Determining a Model for the Mental Hospital.* Wash., D.C.: Amer. Psychiat. Assoc., Comm. Public. Info., Paper No. 131 (Cf. Schwartz, M. S., & Schwartz, C. G., 1959) (I B 1; I C 3; I A 1).

―――― ―――― (1964), *Social Approaches to Mental Health Care.* N.Y.: Columbia Univ. Press (II B 1).

―――― & Schockley, E. L. (1956), *The Nurse and the Mental Patient: A Study of Interpersonal Relations.* N.Y.: Russell Sage Found. (II A 3 g; I C 3).

―――― & Will, G. T. (1953), Low morale and mutual withdrawal on a mental hospital ward. *Psychiatry,* 15:337-353 (I B 1; I C 3; II B 1).

Schwartz, R. A. (1969), The role of family planning in the primary prevention of mental illness. *Amer. J. Psychiat.,* 25:1711-1718 (II B 7).

Scott, D. (1956), Chronic mental patients' reactions to opening their ward. *Amer. J. Psychiat.,* 113:336 (II B 2).

Scott, R. D. (1962), A conceptual model of a hospital as an aid to the everyday handling of psychotic patients. *Psychiatry,* 25:208-218 (I B 1; I C 3; I A 1).

Scully, A. W. (1945), The work of a chaplain in a state hospital for mental disorders. *J. Nerv. Ment. Dis.,* 101:264 (II A 3 k).

Seale, A. L., Miller, M., Watkins, C., & Wurster, C. (1959), Changing nature of state hospital populations. *Dis. Nerv. Syst.,* 20: 530-534 (I A 1).

―――― & Watkins, C. (1958), Recent advances in mental health care by the state mental hospital. *J. La. St. Med. Soc.,* 110:379-383 (I C 3).

Seefeldt, C. J. (1964), Patients' participation at the staff level. In: Role of the psychiatric social worker in mental health programs: A symposium. *J. Psychiat. Soc. Worker,* 13:142 (II B 3; II A 3 f).

Seitz, P. F. D. (1961), Theory and technique in the narcissistic neuroses. Presented to the Chicago Psychoanalytic Society, Oct. 14. (Based upon patients treated at the state hospital reported in the present study.) (I C 3; II C 1).

—— (1962), Selected excerpts from the literature on the use and training of volunteers in mental hospitals. Chicago: Unpublished syllabus, Chicago Inst. Psychoanal. (II A 3 j; II C 1).

—— (1963a), The integration of volunteers in psychiatric teams. Presented at the Annual Awards Day Ceremonies, Chicago State Hospital, May 27 (II A 3 j; II A 2; I B 3; II C 1).

—— (1963b), Report of a training program in group processes — National Education Association. Chicago: Unpublished report to the Chicago Inst. Psychoanal. (I B 3; II C 1).

—— (1964), Freud's contributions to psychiatry. *Ment. Hygiene* 48:74-81 (I C 3; II C 1).

—— , Jacob, E., Koenig, H., Koenig, R., McPherson, W. G., Miller, A. A., Stewart, R. L., & Stock, D. (1963), A coordinated consultant team for remote state hospitals. *Arch. Gen. Psychiat.,* 8:283-288 (II C 3).

Sewall, L. G., (1958), Management principles applied to the mental hospital. *Ment. Hosp.,* 9:42-45 (I B 2).

—— , Brillin, J., & Lebar, F. M. (1955), Through the patient's eyes: Hospital-patient attitudes. *Ment. Hygiene,* 39:284-292 (I B 1; I C 3; II B 3).

Sharp, A. A. (1953), *How Volunteers Work in State Hospitals.* Chicago: Dept. Ment. Health (II A 3 j).

Shattan, S. P. (1966), Group treatment of conditionally discharged patients in a mental health clinic. *Amer. J. Psychiat.,* 122:798-805 (II B 1; II B 5).

Shaw, D., & Samuel, A. (1959), Medical administration in psychiatric hospitals. *Lancet,* 2:170-172 (I B 2).

Shearer, M. L., Cain, A. C., Finch, S. M., et al. (1968), Unexpected effects of an "open door" policy on birth rates of women in state hospitals. *Amer. J. Orthopsychiat.,* 38:413-417 (II B 2).

Sheeley, W. E. (1960), Using the mental hospital for postgraduate education. *GP,* 22:167-171 (II C 1; II B 6).

—— (1961), The nonpsychiatrist physician in psychiatric hospitals or services. Reactions of U.S. psychiatrists. *Ment. Hosp.,* 12:50-52 (II A 3 c; I C 2; I C 1).

Sheffel, I. (1951), Administration — a point of view for psychiatrists. *Bull. Menninger Clin.*, 15:131 (I B 2; I C 2; II A 3 c).

Sheimo, S. L., Paynter, J., & Szurek, S. A. (1949), Problems of staff interaction with spontaneous group formations on a children's psychiatric ward. *Amer. J. Orthopsychiat.*, 19:599-611 (I B 1; I B 3; II B 3).

Sherif, M., & Sherif, C. W. (1956), *An Outline of Social Psychology. Part III: Human Interaction and Its Products: Group Structure and Norms (Values)*. N.Y.: Harper, pp. 119-333 (II B 1).

Sherman, R. W., & Hildreth, A. M. (1970), A resident group process training seminar. *Amer. J. Psychiat.*, 127:372-375 (II B 1; II C 1).

Shotwell, A. M., Dingman, H. F., & Tarjan, G. (1960), Need for improved criteria in evaluating job performance of state hospital employees. *Amer. J. Ment. Defic.*, 65:208-213 (I C 1; II A 3 a).

Shuman, I. (1960), Ex-patients make good volunteers. *Ment. Hosp.*, 11:28-29 (II B 3; II A 3 j).

Silver, R. J., & Sines, L. K. (1963), State hospital and teaching institute treatment results. *Dis. Nerv. Syst.*, 24:414-419 (I C 3; II C 1).

Silverberg, J. W., D'Elia, F. G., Rabiner, E. L., & Gralnick, A. (1964), The implementation of psychoanalytic concepts in hospital practice. In: Masserman, J. H. (Ed.), *Science and Psychoanalysis* 7:280-289. N.Y.: Grune & Stratton (II A 3 b; I C 3; II C 1).

Simmel, E. (1937), The psychoanalytic sanatarium and the psychoanalytic movement. *Bull. Menninger Clin.*, 1:133-143 (II A 3 b; I C 3; II C 1).

Simmons, O. G., Davis, J. A., & Spencer, K. (1956), Structured strains in release from a mental hospital. *Soc. Probs.*, 4:21-28 (II B 5).

Simon, J. L. (1961), Neurology in the mental hospital. *Bol. Assoc. Med. P. Rico.*, 53:1-8 (II A 3 d).

Simpson, G., & Kline, N. S. (1962), A new type psychiatric research ward. *Amer. J. Psychiat.*, 119:511-514 (II C 2).

Singlinger, E., & Faris, M. (1965), Nurse and social worker collaborate in a milieu program. *Nurs. Outlook*, 3:296-298 (II B 1; II A 2; II A 3 g; II A 3 f).

Sivadon, P. (1952), *The Place of the Psychiatric Hospital in the Mental Health Service*. Geneva: World Health Org., MENT, 34 (I A 1; I C 3; II B 6).

Sletten, I. W., & Bennett, H. (1963), A mixed cottage for long-term patients. *Ment. Hosp.,* 14:437 (II B 1).

Small, I. F. (1961), Patient freedom: A view from Michigan. *Amer. J. Psychiat.,* 118:139-141 (II B 2).

———, Matarazzo, R. G., & Small, J. G. (1963), Total ward therapy groups in psychiatric treatment. *Amer. J. Psychother.,* 17:254-265 (II B 1; I C 3).

Smith, C. M. (1971), Crisis and aftermath: Community psychiatry in Saskatchewan, 1963-69. *Canad. Psychiat. Assoc. J.,* 16:65-76 (II B 7).

Smith, H. L. (1949), The sociological study of hospitals. Chicago: Unpublished Ph.D. thesis, Dept. of Sociol., Univ. of Chicago (I B 1).

——— (1957), Professional strains and the hospital context. In: Greenblatt, M., Levinson, D. J., & Williams, R. H. (Eds.) (1957), pp. 9-13 (I B 1; I B 3).

——— & Levinson, D. J. (1957), The major aims and organizational characteristics of mental hospitals. In: Greenblatt, M., Levinson, D. J., & Williams, R. H. (Eds.) (1957), pp. 3-8 (I B 1).

——— & Thrasher, J. (1963), Roles, cliques and sanctions: Dimensions of patient society. *Internat. J. Soc. Psychiat.,* 9:184-191 (I B 1; II B 1).

Smith, J. A., Swanson, D. W., Loomis, S. D., & Beckering, B. (1962), Fifty years in a mental hospital. *JAMA,* 181:750-753 (I A 1; I C 3).

Smith, S., Gibb, G. M., & Martin, A. A. (1960), Metamorphosis of a mental hospital. Application of McKeown's comprehensive unit. *Lancet,* 2:592-593 (II A 1).

——— ——— ——— (1963), Using mental hospitals for other purposes. *Lancet,* 2:398-400 (I A 1; II B 6).

Smith, T. C., Bower, W. H., & Wignell, C. M. (1965), Influence of policy and drugs on Colorado state hospital population. *Arch. Gen. Psychiat.,* 12:352 (I A 1).

Snow, H. B. (1958), The open door hospital. *Canad. J. Pub. Health,* 49:363-369 (II B 2).

——— (1959), Open ward policy at St. Lawrence State Hospital. *Amer. J. Psychiat.,* 115:779-789 (II B 2).

——— (1962a), The open door and the community. *Amer. Pract.,* 13:403-409 (II B 2; II B 6).

——— (1962b), The hospital we opened: Some comments in retrospect. *Ment. Hosp.,* 13:573-579 (II B 2).

Sobin, J. (1959), The general practitioner: A neglected resource for the psychiatric ward. *Med. Times,* 87:910-913 (I C 1; II B 6; II A 3 a).

Social Science Institute (1961), *Research on the Psychiatric Hospital as a Social System.* St. Louis: Social Science Inst., Univ. College, Washington Univ. (I B 1; II C 2).

Sokolov, A. A. (1960), On various prerequisites for organization of scientific work in the area of a psychoneurological hospital. *Zh. Neuropat. Psikhiat. Korsakov.,* 60:1373-1377 (Russian) (II C 2).

Solomon, C. (1959), Report from the asylum. In: Feldman, G., & Gartenberg, M. (Eds.), *The Beat Generation and the Angry Young Men.* N.Y.: Dell, pp. 177-178 (I A 1).

Solomon, H. C. (1960), Hospital psychiatry today. *Ment. Hosp.,* 11:14-17 (I A 1).

Solt, R. I., & Walker, W. H. (1963), State mental and penal hospitals: A source of clinical patients while providing better medical care. *J. Nat. Med. Assoc.,* 55:231-232 (I C 3; II C 1).

Sommer, R. (1958), Occupational therapists as specialists in mental hospitals. *Amer. J. Occup. Ther.,* 12:250-254 (II A 3 h; I C 3).

———— (1959a), Studies in personal space. *Sociometry,* 22:247-260 (I B 1; I A 1).

———— (1959b), Patients who grow old in a mental hospital. *Geriatrics,* 14:586-587 (I A 1; I C 3).

Souelem, O. (1955), Mental patients' attitudes toward mental hospitals. *J. Clin. Psychol.,* 11:181-185 (II B 3; I B 1).

Spiegel, J. P. (1957), The resolution of role conflicts within the family. *Psychiatry,* 20:1-16 (II B 4).

Srole, L., Langner, T., Michael, S., et al. (1962), *Mental Health in the Metropolis: The Midtown Manhattan Project.* Vol. I. N.Y.: McGraw-Hill (I A 1).

———— & Schrijvers, J. (1968), Gheel, Belgium: The prototype therapeutic community. Presented at the Annual Meeting of the American Psychiatric Association, Boston, May 13-17 (II B 1; II B 7).

Stainbrook, E. (1955a), Human action in the social system of the psychiatric hospital. In: *Better Social Services for Mentally Ill Patients.* N.Y.: Amer. Assoc. Psychiat. Soc. Workers, pp. 1-19 (I B 1).

———— (1955b), The hospital as a therapeutic community. *Neuropsychiat.,* 3:69-87 (II B 1).

Stanton, A. H. (1954), Psychiatric theory and institutional context. *Psychiatry,* 17:19-26 (I B 1).

———— (1957), Problems in analysis of therapeutic implications of the institutional milieu. In: *Symposium on Preventive and Social Psychiatry.* Wash., D.C.: Walter Reed Army Inst. Res., p. 499 (II B 1; I C 3; I B 1; II C 2).

———— & Schwartz, M. S. (1949a), The management of a type of institutional participation in mental illness. *Psychiatry,* 12:13-26 (I B 1).

———— ———— (1949b), Medical opinion and the social context in the mental hospital. *Psychiatry,* 12:243-249 (I C 2; I B 1).

———— ———— (1954), *The Mental Hospital.* N.Y.: Basic Books (I B 1; I C 3).

Steiman, L. A., & Hunt, R. C. (1961), A day care center in a state hospital. *Amer. J. Psychiat.,* 117:1109-1112 (II B 5).

Stein, R. F. (1964), The nursing instructor as model and preceptor. *Ment. Hosp.,* 15:28-32 (II A 3 g; II C 1).

Stein, W. W. (1963), Patterns of a Peruvian mental hospital. *Internat. J. Soc. Psychiat.,* 9:208-215 (I A 1; I C 3).

Stengel, E. (1948), The application of psychoanalytic principles to the hospital in-patient. *J. Ment. Sci.,* 94:773-781 (II A 3 b; I C 3).

Stern, B. E., & Stern, E. S. (1963), Efficiency of mental hospitals. *Brit. J. Prev. Soc. Med.,* 17:11-120 (I A 1).

Sterns, E. M. (1953), *The Attendants Guide.* N.Y.: Nat. Assoc. Ment. Health (II A 3 i).

Stetson, E. R. (1951), The role played by volunteers in a mental hospital. *Amer. J. Occup. Ther.,* 5:203 (II A 3 j).

Stevenson, G. S. (1942), *Ideals and Principles for Proper Management of the Mentally Ill.* N.Y.: Nat. Assoc. Ment. Health (I C 3; I A 1).

Stewart, R. L., Jacob, E., Koenig, H., Koenig, R., McPherson, W. G., Miller, A. A., Seitz, P. F. D., & Stock, D. (1963), The state hospital consultant team as an educational instrument. In: Masserman, J. (Ed.), *Current Psychiatric Therapies* 3:264-271. N.Y.: Grune & Stratton (II C 3; II C 1).

Stokes, A. B. (1961), The provision for appropriate aftercare: Hospital and community collaboration. *Ment. Hosp.,* 12:36-38 (II B 5; II B 6).

Stone, O. M. (1961), The three worlds of the back yard. *Ment. Hygiene,* 45:18-27 (I B 1).

Stotland, E., & Kohler, A. L. (1965), *Life and Death of a Mental Hospital*. Seattle: Univ. of Wash. Press (I B 2; I B 1; I A 1).

Stotsky, B. A., Sacks, J. M., & Daston, P. G. (1956), Predicting the work performance of psychiatric aides by psychological tests. *J. Consult. Psychol.*, 3:193-199 (II A 3 j).

Strauss, A., & Sabshin, M. (1961), Large state mental hospitals—social values, societal resources. *Arch. Gen. Psychiat.*, 5:565-577 (I A 1; I C 1; II B 6).

——— , Schatzman, L., Buder, R., et al. (1964), *Psychiatric Ideologies and Institutions*. N.Y.: Free Press (I A 1).

Strickler, M. (1965), Applying crisis theory in a walk-in clinic. *Soc. Casework*, 3:150-154 (II B 7).

Stringham, J. A. (1952), Rehabilitating chronic psychiatric patients. *Amer. J. Psychiat.*, 108:924 (I C 3; I A 1; I B 2).

Strodtbeck, F. L., & Hare, A. P. (1954), Bibliography of small group research (from 1900 through 1953). *Sociometry*, 17:107-178 (II C 2; II B 1).

Strune, M., & Hahn, A. (1949), The nursing team in the hospital. *Amer. J. Nurs.*, 49:5-11 (II A 3 g; II A 2).

Stubbins, J., & Soloman, L. (1959), Patient government . . . a case study. *Ment. Hygiene*, 43:539-544 (II B 3).

Stubblebine, J. M., & Decker, J. (1971), Are urban mental health centers worth it? *Amer. J. Psychiat.*, 127:908-912 (II B 7).

Surber, G. P., & Niswander, G. D. (1959), Patient interaction on admission wards. *Ment. Hosp.*, 10:22 (II B 3; I B 1).

Szurek, S. A. (1947), Dynamics of staff interaction in hospital psychiatric treatment of children. *Amer. J. Orthopsychiat.*, 17:652-664 (I B 1).

——— (1951), The family and the staff in hospital psychiatric therapy of children. *Amer. J. Orthopsychiat.*, 21:597-611 (II B 4).

Taggart, D. (1953), What shall be taught—designed occupational therapy for the psychiatric team. *Amer. J. Psychiat.*, 110:171-174 (II A 3 h; II A 3; II C 1).

Tallman, F. F. (1959), *The State Mental Hospital in Transition*. Wash., D.C.: Amer. Psychiat. Assoc., Comm. Public Info., Paper No. 133 (I A 1; I C 3).

——— (1960), The state hospital in transition. *Amer. J. Psychiat.*, 116:818-824 (I A 1).

Tarjan, G. (1964), The administrator's responsibilities toward research. *Ment. Hosp.*, 15:620-628 (II C 2; I B 2).

Tarumianz, M. A. (1960), The "open door" for mental patients. *Delaware Med. J.*, 32:411-414 (II B 2).

Tarwater, J. S. (1960), Psychiatric treatment in a mental hospital. *Dis. Nerv. Syst.*, 21:289-291 (I C 3).

Taube, C. A. (1973), *Utilization of Mental Health Facilities*. Wash., D.C.: Dept. HEW, Public. No. NIH-74-657, Mental Health Statistics Series B, No. 5 (I A 1).

Taxel, H. (1953), Authority structure in a mental hospital ward. Chicago: Unpublished Master's thesis. Dept. of Sociol., Univ. of Chicago. (I B 1; I B 2; I C 2).

Teplinsky, J. (1963), Adjunctive therapies in the treatment of mental illness. *Hosp. Manag.*, 95:64-67 (II A 3).

Terhune, W. (1957), Administrative psychiatry: A new field — challenging and rewarding. *Amer. J. Psychiat.*, 114:64-67 (I B 2).

Thale, T. (1962), Public psychiatric hospitals. *Hosp. Progr.*, 43:80-83 (I A 1; I C 3).

Thelen, H. A. (1954), *Dynamics of Groups at Work*. Chicago: Univ. of Chicago Press (See esp. Chaps. 3, 10, & 11.) (II B 1).

Thomson, C. P. (1970), Involving the private sector in community psychiatry. *Amer. J. Psychiat.*, 127:363-368 (II B 7).

———— & Bell, N. W. (1969), Evaluation of a rural community mental health program. *Arch. Gen. Psychiat.*, 20:448-456 (II B 7).

Thurston, J. (1951), The patients rule themselves. *Smith Coll. Stud. Soc. Work*, 22:27-51 (II B 3).

Tietz, E. G., & Grotjahn, M. (1951), Psychiatric team work — an integrated therapy. *JAMA*, 174:1055-1059 (II A 2; I C 3).

Tischler, G. L., & Riedel, D. C. (1973), A criterion approach to patient care evaluation. *Amer. J. Psychiat.*, 130:913-915 (I C 3).

Todd, G. S., & Wittkower, E. (1948), The psychological aspects of sanatorium management. *Lancet*, 1:49-53 (I B 2; I C 3).

Tolor, A. (1962), The personality need structure of psychiatric attendants. *Ment. Hygiene*, 46:218-222 (II A 3 i).

Toobert, S., Scott, F. G., & Lewis, J. D. (1962), Relation of various indicators of ward management to measures of staff attitudes in a large mental hospital. *J. Health Hum. Behav.*, 3:185-193 (I B 1; I C 2).

Toomey, L. C., Reznikoff, M., Brady, J. P., & Schumann, D. W. (1961), Attitudes of nursing students toward psychiatric treatment and hospitals. *Ment. Hygiene*, 45:589-602 (II A 3 g; I C 3; II C 1).

Tooth, G. C., & Brooke, E. M. (1961), Trends in mental hospital population and their effect on future planning. *Lancet* (April 1):710-713 (I A 1).

Torrey, E. F. (1969), The case for the indigenous therapist. *Arch. Gen. Psychiat.,* 20:365-373 (II B 7).

Tucker, G. J., & Maxmen, J. S. (1973), The practice of hospital psychiatry: A formulation. *Amer. J. Psychiat.,* 130:887-891 (I C 3).

Tuckman, J., & Lavell, M. (1960), Effect of removal of overcrowding on patient movement. *Ment. Hygiene,* 44:269-273 (I A 1).

Tudor, G. E. (1952), A sociopsychiatric nursing approach to intervention in a problem of mutual withdrawal on a mental hospital ward. *Psychiatry,* 15:193-217 (II A 3 g; I B 1).

Ullman, L. P., & Gurel, L. (1964), Staffing and psychiatric hospital effectiveness. *Arch. Gen. Psychiat.,* 11:360-367 (I C 1).

Urbaitis, J. C. (Mod.) (1975), New mental health teams. Presented to the Annual Meeting of the American Psychiatric Association, Anaheim, Calif., May 5-9. *Scientific Proceedings in Summary Form.* Wash., D.C.: Amer. Psychiat. Assoc., p. 309 (II A 2).

Vail, D. J. (1959), Medical or non-medical superintendency? *Ment. Hosp.,* 10:9-12 (I B 2).

———— (1964), Facets of institutional living: The danger of dehumanization. *Ment. Hosp.,* 15:599-601 (I A 1; II B 1).

Van Dusen, W., Klatte, E., & Wilson, W. (1963), Nonmedical unit administration. *Ment. Hosp.,* 14:483-486 (I C 2; I B 2; II A 1).

———— & Rector, W. (1963), A Q Sort study of the ideal administrator. *J. Clin. Psychol.,* 19:244 (I B 2).

Vaughan, W. T., Jr., & Field, M. G. (1963), New perspectives of mental patient care. *Amer. J. Public Health,* 53:237-242 (I C 3).

Victoroff, V. M. (1969), *Hospitalizing the Mentally Ill in Ohio.* Cleveland: Case Western Reserve Univ. Press (I A 1).

Vitale, J. H. (1961), The therapeutic community: A review article. In: *Research on the Psychiatric Hospital as a Social System.* St. Louis: Social Science Inst., Univ. College, Washington Univ. Also in: Wessen, A. F. (1964), pp. 91-110 (II B 1; II C 2).

Wachpress, M. (1972), Goals and functions of the community mental health center. *Amer. J. Psychiat.,* 129:187-190 (II B 7).

Wade, D. (1941), Occupational therapy as a component of a unified treatment program in psychiatry. *Occup. Ther.,* 20:167-175 (II A 3 h; II A 2; I C 3).

Wadeson, R. W. (Reporter) (1975), Psychoanalysis and community psychiatry: Reflections on some theoretical implications. *J. Amer. Psychoanal. Assoc.,* 23:177-189 (II A 3 b; II B 7).

Wake, F. R. (1959), The open door philosophy: A concept of free-dom. *Med. Serv. J. Canada,* 15:551-560 (II B 2).

———— (1961), Some observations on the "open door" in Canadian and other hospitals. *Canad. Psychiat. Assoc. J.,* 6:96-102 (II B 2).

Wales, B. G. (1960), Rewards of illness. Observations on institu-tionalization by a former neuropsychiatric patient. *Ment. Hygiene,* 44:55-63 (I B 1; I C 3).

Walker, W. R., Parsons, L. B., & Skelton, W. D. (1973), Brief hospitalization on a crisis service: A study of patient and treat-ment variables. *Amer. J. Psychiat.,* 130:896-899 (I C 3).

Walkiewicz, S. T. (1946), Convalescent patients as mental hospital employees. *Smith Coll. Stud. Soc. Work,* 16:282 (II B 3).

Wallace, S. E. (Ed.) (1971), *Total Institutions.* Chicago: Aldine (I A 1).

Wanklin, J. M., Fleming, D. F., Buck, C., & Hobbs, G. E. (1956), Discharge and readmission among mental hospital patients; cohort analysis. *AMA Arch. Neurol. Psychiat.,* 76:660-669 (I A 1).

Ward, M. J. (1955), *The Snake Pit.* N.Y.: New Amer. Library (I A 1; I C 3).

Wayne, G. J. (1961a), Two roads to treatment. I. The case for the psychiatric hospital. *Ment. Hosp.,* 12:5-10 (I C 3; II B 2).

———— (1961b), An evaluation of new trends in psychiatric hos-pitals. *Ment. Hosp.,* 13:10-15 (I A 1; I C 3).

Wechsler, H. (1960), The self-help organization in the mental health field: Recovery, Inc., a case study. *J. Nerv. Ment. Dis.,* 130:297-314 (II B 3; II B 5).

———— (1961), Transitional residences for former mental patients: A survey of half-way houses and related rehabilitation facilities. *Ment. Hygiene,* 45:67 (II B 5; II B 6).

————, Grosser, G. H., & Greenblatt, M. (1965), Research evalu-ating antidepressant medications on hospitalized mental patients: A survey of published reports during a five-year period. *J. Nerv. Ment. Dis.,* 141:231-239 (II C 2).

Weinberg, S. K. (1952), *Society and Personality Disorders.* N.Y.: Prentice-Hall (I B 1; II B 6).

Weinstein, A. S., DiPasquale, D., & Winsor, F. (1973), Relation-ships between length of stay in and out of the New York state mental hospitals. *Amer. J. Psychiat.,* 130:904-909 (I C 3).

———— & Patton, R. E. (1970), Trends in "chronicity" in the New

York state mental hospitals. *Amer. J. Public Health,* 60:1071-1080 (I A 1; I C 3).

Weintraub, W. (1964), "The VIP syndrome": A clinical study in hospital psychiatry. *J. Nerv. Ment. Dis.,* 138:181-193 (I B 1; I C 3; I B 2).

Weiss, P., Macaulay, J., & Pincus, A. (1966), Geographic factors and the release of patients from state mental hospitals. *Amer. J. Psychiat.,* 123:408-412 (I A 1).

Wessen, A. F. (1951), The social structure of a modern hospital. New Haven: Unpublished Ph.D. thesis, Dept. of Sociol., Yale Univ. (I B 1).

—— (1964), *The Psychiatric Hospital as a Social System.* Springfield: Ill.: Charles C Thomas (I B 1).

West, L. J. (1973), The future of psychiatric education. *Amer. J. Psychiat.,* 130:521-528 (II C 1).

Wheatley, J. (1963a), Psychiatric nursing. Patients working for pay. *Nurs. Times,* 59:662 (II B 3; II A 3 g).

—— (1963b), Patients working for pay—further comments. *Nurs. Times,* 59:1067-1068 (II B 3; II A 3 g).

Whitaker, D. S., & Lieberman, M. A. (1964), *Psychotherapy Through the Group Process.* N.Y.: Atherton (Prentice-Hall) (II B 1).

White, R. R. (1943), The social services in the state hospitals of Illinois. *Ment. Hygiene,* 27:554 (II A 3 f).

Whitehorn, J. C., Braceland, F. J., Lippard, V. W., & Malamud, W. (Eds.) (1953), *The Psychiatrist—His Training and Development.* Wash., D.C.: Amer. Psychiat. Assoc. (II A 3 c; II C 1).

Whitely, R. (1960), Australian day hospital. *Med. J. Austral.,* 2:728-731 (II B 5).

Whitman, J. R., & Duffey, R. F. (1961), The relationship between type of therapy received and a patient's perception of his illness. *J. Nerv. Ment. Dis.,* 133:288-292 (I B 1; I B 3).

Whitman, R. M. (1956), The rating and group dynamics of the psychiatric staff conference. *Psychiatry,* 19:333-340 (I B 1; II B 1).

Whitmer, C. A., & Conover, C. G. (1959), A study of critical incidents in the hospitalization of the mentally ill. *Soc. Work,* 40:89-94 (I B 1).

Wilder, J. F., Karasu, B., & Kligler, D. (1972), The hospital "dumping syndrome": Causes and treatment. *Amer. J. Psychiat.,* 128:1446-1449 (I A 1).

Wilkins, G. D., Lea, R. V., Nicholson, A. L., Oldmeadow, D. J., & Richards, W. R. (1963), A therapeutic community development in a state psychiatric hospital. *Med. J. Austral.,* 2:220-224 (II B 1).

Will, G. T. (1957), Psychiatric nursing administration and its implications for patient care. In: Greenblatt, M., Levinson, D. J., & Williams, R. H. (Eds.) (1957), pp. 237-247 (II A 3 g; I B 2; I C 3).

Williams, J. H., & Williams, H. M. (1961), Attitudes toward mental illness, anomia and authoritarianism among state hospital nursing students and attendants. *Ment. Hygiene,* 45:418-424 (II A 3 g; II A 3 i; I B 2; I B 1).

Williams, R. H. (1957), The movement from custodial hospital to therapeutic community: Implications for theory. In: Greenblatt, M., Levinson, D. J., & Williams, R. H. (Eds.) (1957), pp. 620-632 (II B 1; I C 3; I B 1; I B 2).

—————— & Ozarin, L. D. (Eds.) (1968), *Community Mental Health: An International Perspective.* San Francisco: Jossey-Bass (II B 7).

Williams, T. G. (1960), Problems in the team treatment of adults in state mental hospitals. Panel, 1958. 2. Possible effects of the introduction of team treatment into state hospitals. *Amer. J. Orthopsychiat.,* 30:95-99 (II A 2; I B 3; I C 3).

Wilmer, H. A. (1958a), *Social Psychiatry in Action.* Springfield, Ill.: Charles C Thomas (II B 1).

—————— (1958b), Toward a definition of the therapeutic community. *Amer. J. Psychiat.,* 114:824-833 (II B 1).

Wilson, E., & Bartlett, H. M. (1955), Referrals from hospital to social agencies: Some principles and problems. *Soc. Casework,* 36:457-465 (II B 5; II B 6).

Wing, J. K. (1962), Institutionalism in mental hospitals. *Brit. J. Soc. Clin. Psychol.,* 1:38-51 (I C 3; I B 1).

—————— (1963), Rehabilitation of psychiatric patients. *Brit. J. Psychiat.,* 109:635-641 (I C 3).

Winston, N. T., Jr. (1964), Tennessee's new state hospital minimizes institutional routines. *Ment. Hosp.,* 15:628-630 (I B 2; I C 3; I B 1).

Wise, H. B., Torrey, E. F., McDade, A., et al. (1968), The family health worker. *Amer. J. Public Health,* 58:1828-1836 (II B 6; II B 7).

Wisebord, N., Denbar, H. C., Charatan, F. B., & Travis, J. H. (1958), Patient reactions to the open door. *Amer. J. Psychiat.,* 115:518-521 (II B 2; I C 3; I B 1).

Wolfe, H. E. (1962), A two year analysis of an in-hospital vocational rehabilitation program. *Dis. Nerv. Syst.,* 23:640-641 (II A 3 h; I C 3).

Wolff, K. (1960), The volunteer as a member of the psychiatric team. *Ment. Hygiene,* 44:206-209 (II A 3 j; II A 2).

Wolford, J. A. (1975), Involuntary hospitalization: A logical compromise? Presented to the Annual Meeting of the American Psychiatric Association, Anaheim, Calif., May 5-9. *Scientific Proceedings in Summary Form.* Wash., D.C.: Amer. Psychiat. Assoc., pp. 147-148 (I C 3; II B 2).

Wolfrom, E., Pang, L. L., & Courtney, E. M. (1963), Roads to the mental hospital. *Ment. Hygiene,* 47:398-407 (II B 6; I A 1).

Wood, E. C., Rakusin, J. M., & Morse, E. (1960), Interpersonal aspects of psychiatric hospitalization. I. The Admission. *Arch. Gen. Psychiat.,* 3:641 (I B 1; I C 3; I A 1).

———— ———— ———— (1962), Interpersonal aspects of psychiatric hospitalization. II. Some correlations between the admission circumstances and the hospital treatment experience. III. The follow-up survey. *Arch. Gen. Psychiat.,* 6:39-45; 46-55 (I B 1; I C 3; I A 1).

Wood, P. E. (1975), Family therapy in aftercare: A unique approach. Presented to the Annual Meeting of the American Psychiatric Association, Anaheim, Calif., May 5-9. *Scientific Proceedings in Summary Form.* Wash., D.C.: Amer. Psychiat. Assoc., p. 24 (II B 4; II B 5).

Worden, F. (1951), Psychotherapeutic aspects of authority. *Psychiatry,* 14:9-10 (I B 2; I C 2; I C 3).

World Health Organization (1953), *Expert Committee on Mental Health—Third Report.* Geneva: WHO, Technical Report, Series No. 73 (I C 3; I A 1).

Wynne, L. (1958), Pseudo-mutuality in the family relations of schizophrenics. *Psychiatry,* 21:205-220 (II B 4).

Yolles, S. F., et al. (1967), Community psychiatry. *Amer. J. Psychiat.,* 124 (Suppl.):1-76 (II B 7).

Young, C. L. (1959), A therapeutic community with an open door in a psychiatric receiving service. *Arch. Neurol. Psychiat.,* 81:335-340 (II B 1; II B 2; I C 3).

Zander, A., Cohen, A. E., & Stolland, E. (1957), *Role Relations in the Mental Health Professions.* Ann Arbor, Mich.: Research Center for Group Dynamics, Univ. of Mich. (I B 1; I B 3).

Zaslove, M. O., Ungerleider, J. T., & Fuller, M. C. (1966), How psychiatric hospitalization helps: Patient views *vs.* staff views. *J. Nerv. Ment. Dis.,* 142:568-576 (I C 3; II B 3).

Zee, H. J. (1962), The patient's responsibility: Reasons for its neglect in psychiatric hospital treatment. *Bull. Menninger Clin.,* 26: 299-308 (II B 3; I C 3).

Zeitlyn, B. B. (1967), The therapeutic community: Fact or fantasy. *Brit. J. Psychiat.,* 113:1083-1086 (II B 1).

Zimmerman, W. A., & Appleby, L. (1959), Research in state mental hospitals. I. The research milieu. Presented to Kansas and Southwest Psychological Associations, Topeka, April (II C 2).

Zubowicz, G. (1959), Rx for reorganization. *Ment. Hosp.,* 10(3):35-36 (I B 2; I B 1).

_____ (1963), The change to a unit system. *Psychiatric Studies and Projects,* No. 8. Wash., D.C.: Amer. Psychiat. Assoc. (II A 1).

Zwerling, I. (1963), Applied psychoanalysis in community psychiatry. Presented to Alumni Association of Columbia University Psychoanalytic Clinic, April 19 (II A 3 b; II B 7).

_____ & Coleman, M. D. (1959), Psychiatric emergency clinic: Flexible way of meeting community mental health needs. *Amer. J. Psychiat.,* 115:980-984 (II B 7).

_____ & Wilder, J. (1962), Day hospital treatment for acutely psychotic patients. In: Masserman, J. (Ed.), *Current Psychiatric Therapies,* 2:200-210. N.Y.: Grune & Stratton (II B 5).

Subject Index

Problems of state hospital psychiatry.
A. Problems of largeness and isolation.
  1. *Statistics, surveys, critiques, and forecasts:*
  Adams (1961), Albee & Dickey (1957), Amer. Hosp. Assoc.
  (1945-75), Amer. Psychiat. Assoc. (1950a), (1951a),
  (1952), (1962), (1969), (1971), (1974), Anon. (1936),
  Baker, A. (1963), Baker, E. (1960), Barton (1962), (1963),
  Barton et al. (1962), Belknap (1956), Bickford (1963),
  Blain (1949), (1963), Blain et al. (1963), Bloomberg &
  Rockmore (1967), Bond (1947), (1956), Bonner, C. &
  Taylor (1939), Braceland (1956), Braginsky et al. (1969),
  Brill (1975a), (1975b), Brill & Patton (1962), (1964),
  Brooke (1962), (1963), Brown, G. (1960), Brown G. et al.
  (1961), Bunker (1944), Burdock et al. (1961), Bureau of
  Census (1941), Bush (1959a), Canad. Ment. Health Assoc.
  (1962), Chu & Trotter (1974), Clayton (1974), Colman &
  Greenblatt (1963), Council of State Govts. (1950), (1953),
  Davidson (1959), Davidson & Russell (1963), Davis, J. A.
  et al. (1957), Dept. HEW (1960), Deutsch (1949), Doehme
  et al. (1964), Dunham & Meltzer (1946), Ed. Comment
  (1963), Ewalt et al. (1960), Fein (1958), Feldman, P.
  (1952), Gammon (1950), Gerty (1963), Goldberg, A. &
  Rubin (1964), Gore & Jones (1961), Gorman (1963),
  Goshen (1961), Greenblatt (1975), Grimes (1951), (1954),
  Grob (1966), (1973), GAP (1948b), (1949), (1950), (1953),
  (1961c), (1964), (1969), Gurel (1964), Hall (1962), Hamilton, S. (1944), Hammersley & Vosburgh (1967), Hansell &
  Hart (1970), Hobbs et al. (1965), Hollingshead & Redlich
  (1958), Holzberg (1960), Houck (1975), Hunt (1960), Hurd

237

et al. (1916), Jackson, J. (1964), Jaffary (1942), Johnson, D.
& Dodds (1957), Joint Commiss. Ment. Illness & Health
(1961), Joint Info. Serv. APA & NAMH (1960), Jones, K.
(1955), Jones, K. et al. (1961), Jones, M. & Tuxford (1963),
Kanno et al. (1974), Kanno & Scheidemandel (1970),
Kerkhoff (1952), Kingston (1963), Kramer, M. (1957),
Kramer, M. et al. (1955), Kraus (1957), Kremens (1962),
Kubie (1968), Langsley et al. (1973), Lazarus et al. (1963),
Lehrman (1960), Letemandia & Harris (1974), Levinson
(1964), Leyberg (1959), Locke et al. (1958), Macht (1975),
Macinnes & Macaulay (1963), Mackie (1963), MacKinnon
(1963), Maddison (1960), Maine (1947), Malzberg (1953),
Mangum (1963), Maxmen et al. (1974), Mechanick &
Nathan (1965), Med. Assoc. Ga. (1959), Menninger, W.
C. (1942), Mercier (1894), Mishler & Wexler (1963),
Morgan, R. & Cook (1963), Murphy, B. (1951), Nat.
Inst. Ment. Health (1969), (1972), (1974), Newcomb
(1961), Nurnberger (1961), O'Dea (1961), Odegard
(1968), Ozarin & Levenson (1969), Ozarin & Taube (1974),
Parkes (1963), Pasamanick (1959), Person (1962), Public
Health Serv. (1947), (1953), Pugh & MacMahon (1962),
Puthu (1959), Rees & Glatt (1956), Reich (1973), Robinson,
R. et al. (1963), Ropschitz (1963), Rose (1955), Rowell
(1955), Rutman & Egan (1975), Schulberg & Baker (1975),
Schwartz, M. & Schwartz (1959), (1960), Scott, R. (1962),
Seale et al. (1959), Sivadon (1952), Smith, J. et al. (1962),
Smith, S. et al. (1963), Smith, T. et al. (1965), Soloman, C.
(1959), Soloman, H. (1960), Sommer (1959a), (1959b),
Srole et al. (1962), Stein, W. (1963), Stern & Stern (1963),
Stevenson (1942), Stotland & Kohler (1965), Strauss et al.
(1964), Strauss & Sabshin (1961), Stringham (1952), Tall-
man (1959), (1960), Taube (1973), Thale (1962), Tooth &
Brooke (1961), Tuckman & Lavell (1960), Vail (1964),
Victoroff (1969), Wallace (1971), Wanklin et al. (1956),
Ward (1955), Wayne (1961b), Weinstein & Patton (1970),
Weiss et al. (1966), Wilder et al. (1972), Wolford et al.
(1972), Wolfrom et al. (1963), Wood E. et al. (1960),
(1962), World Health Org. (1953).

2. *Isolation—as it applies to both patients and staff:*
Albee & Dickey (1957), Amer. Hosp. Assoc. (1945-75),
Batey & Julian (1963), Bloomberg & Rockmore (1967),
Braceland (1962), Conte (1960), Dept. HEW (1954)

Klopfer et al. (1956), Kolb (1962), Kraus (1957), Landy (1961), Lefton et al. (1960), Leighton (1955), Leipold et al. (1964), Lemert (1951), Loeb (1956), (1957), Lundstedt (1965), Main (1946), Marshall & Schlesinger (1949), Martin, H. (1962), McLary (1961), Mercier (1894), von Mering & King (1957a), Middleton (1953), Mishler & Trapp (1956), Morimoto (1955), Murphy, B. (1951), Murray & Cohen (1959), Opler (1956), Parker (1959), Parsons (1952), (1957), Perlin (1960), Perry & Shea (1957), Pinsker et al. (1972), Pishkin & Dredge (1963), Polansky et al. (1950), (1957), Pratt et al. (1960), Rees (1957), Rees & Glatt (1955), Retznikoff et al. (1959a), Rice et al. (1963), Roberts & Lindsay (1962), Rosengren (1961), Rowland (1938), (1939a), Ruesch & Bareson (1949), Rushing (1964), Sabagh et al. (1963), Scher & Johnson (1963), Schneider (1963), Schwartz, C. (1953), Schwartz, C. et al. (1951), Schwartz, M. (1957a), Schwartz, M. & Schwartz (1959), (1960), Schwartz, M. & Will (1953), Scott, R. (1962), Sewall et al. (1955), Sheimo et al. (1949), Smith, H. (1949), (1957), Smith, H. & Levinson (1957), Smith, H. & Thrasher (1963), Soc. Sci. Inst. (1961), Sommer (1959a), Soulem (1955), Stainbrook (1955), Stanton & Schwartz (1949a), (1949b), (1954), Stanton (1954), (1957), Stone (1961), Stotland & Kohler (1965), Surber & Niswander (1959), Szurek (1947), Taxel (1953), Toobert et al. (1962), Tudor (1952), Wales (1960), Weinberg (1952), Weintraub (1964), Wessen (1951), (1964), Whitman, J. & Duffey (1961), Whitman, R. (1956), Whitmer & Conover (1959), Williams, J. & Williams (1961), Williams, R. (1957), Wing (1962), Winston (1964), Wisebord et al. (1958), Wood, E. et al. (1960), (1962), Zubowicz (1959).

2. *Monolithic, authoritarian, administrative structure:*
Adams (1961), Adorno et al. (1950), Amer. Hosp. Assoc. (1945-75), Amer. Psychiat. Assoc. (1946b), Argyris (1962), Baganz (1951), (1953), Barton (1962a), Baur (1957), Bavelas (1948), Belknap (1956), Blake & Mouton (1963), Bosworth (1959), Bravos (1959), Bryan (1936), Bullard (1952), Bush (1960a), Cameron, J. (1963), Capoore et al. (1960), Cartwright (1959), Caudill (1956), Christie, P. (1962), Christie, R. & Jahoda (1954), Clark (1960), (1963), Cook (1960), Cumming, E. et al. (1956), Cumming, E. & Cumming (1956), Duval (1950), (1957), Dykens (1960),

Dykens et al. (1964), Edelson, D. (1960), Ed. Comment (1959b), Ewalt (1956), Fitzsimmons (1950), Fuller (1954), Garber (1958), (1964), Garcia (1960), Gartenberg (1959), Gilbert, D. & Levinson (1956), Goffman (1961), Greenblatt et al. (1957), Greenblatt & Levinson (1959), GAP (1953), (1961a), (1963), Hamburg (1957), Hayes (1959), Haythorn et al. (1956), Heninger (1963), Henry (1954), (1957), (1964), Hoffman (1957), Hutchinson (1963), Hyde et al. (1956), Hyde & Soloman (1951), Jacques (1948), Jones, G. & Waldrum (1960), Jones, M. & Rapoport (1955), Jones, M. & Tuxford (1963), Kahne (1959), Kennard (1957), Laughlin (1954), Levine, J. & Butler (1952), Lundstedt (1965), Martin, H. (1962), May & Wilkinson (1963), McLary (1961), Med. Assoc. Ga. (1959), Mercier (1894), Modlin (1951), Myers & Smith (1959), (1961), (1963), Noroian (1962), Overholser (1939), (1953), Owen (1962), Perkins, C. (1950), Pinsker et al. (1972), Public Health Serv. (1953), Rapoport & Skellern (1957), Ray, I. (1873), Redl (1942), Rubenstein & Lasswell (1966), Rushing (1964), Russell, (1949), Ryniker (1962), Sewall (1958), Shaw & Samuel (1959), Sheffel (1951), Stotland & Kohler (1965), Stringham (1952), Tarjan (1964), Taxel (1953), Terhune (1957), Todd & Wittkower (1948), Vail (1959), Van Dusen et al. (1963), Van Dusen & Rector (1963), Weintraub (1964), Will, G. (1957), Williams, J. & Williams (1961), Williams, R. (1957), Winston (1964), Worden (1951), Zubowicz (1959).

3. *Lack of interdisciplinary communication and collaboration:* Amer. Hosp. Assoc, (1945-75), Argyris (1962), Baker, F. & Schulberg (1967), Baldwin (1963), Bartemeier (1952), Bavelas (1948), Bierer & Haldane (1941), Bishop & Zubowicz (1963), Blake & Mouton (1962), (1963), Borsch (1963), Bovard (1951), Bradford (1953), (1961), (1963), Bradford et al. (1964), Brown, E. (1957), Cameron, J. (1963), Cartwright & Zander (1953), Caudill & Stainbrook (1954), Clancey & Osmond (1959), Crawshaw (1958), Davis, J. E. & Tolor (1959), Denbar (1963), Dickson (1949), Dunlop (1947), Duval (1950), Edelson, M. (1964), Eichorn & Hyde (1950), Eisen et al. (1963), Ewalt (1953), Fitzsimmons (1950), Forman (1951), Gertz (1963), Hamburg (1957), Haythorn et al. (1956), Hjelholt & Miles (1963), Holzberg (1960), Hunt (1960), Jacques (1948), Jones M. & Rapoport (1957),

Kramer, C. (1964), Laughlin (1954), Levine, J. & Butler (1952), Lind & Gralnick (1963), Lubach et al. (1963), Luft (1963), Mann (1959), Margolis et al. (1963), Marshall & Schlesinger (1949), Martin, H. (1962), Miles (1959), (1962), Modlin (1951), Modlin & Faris (1956), Myers (1951), Padula (1960), Peplau (1960), Preston (1948), Redl (1942), Ress & Glatt (1955), Rickman (1950), Rothaus et al. (1963), Rushing (1964), Schwartz, M. (1960), Seitz (1963a), (1963b), Sheimo et al. (1949), Smith, H. (1957), Whitman, J. & Duffey (1961), Williams, T. (1960).

C. Problems of patient care and treatment.

1. *Manpower shortages—in both numbers and skills of staff:*
Albee & Dickey (1957), Amer. Hosp. Assoc. (1945-75), Baer (1952), Blank (1964), Cumming, E. & Cumming (1957a), Dept. HEW (1954), Downing (1958), Dykens (1963), Ed. Comment (1959a), (1959e), (1959f), Edwalds (1962), Eichert (1944), Fink & Zerof (1971), Gaede (1962), Goldberg, A. & Rubin (1964), Goshen (1961), Graham, T. & Zingery (1961), GAP (1948b), Hagopian (1963), Ham (1961), Hoch & Rado (1961), Hunt (1960), Kanno & Scheidemandel (1970), Kline (1950), Kurland & Nilsson (1961), Nat. Assoc. Ment. Health (1960), Nat. Inst. Ment. Health (1972), Newcomb (1961), Sheeley (1961), Shotwell et al. (1960), Sobin (1959), Strauss & Sabshin (1961), Ullman & Gurel (1964).

2. *Weakness of clinical leadership:*
Amer. Hosp. Assoc. (1945-75), Argyris (1962), Bush (1959b), Cartwright (1959), Chessick et al. (1959), Coleman (1950), Cook (1960), Cowen & Schwartz (1960), Cruvant (1953), Cumming, E. & Cumming (1956), Davis, F. (1960), Duval (1950), Dykens (1960), Edwalds (1962), Goffman (1961), Hayes (1959), Haythorn et al. (1956), Henry (1954), (1957), (1964), Hyde et al. (1956), Hyde & Soloman (1951), Jones, M. & Rapoport (1957), Kartus & Schlesinger (1957), Menninger, K. (1949), Menninger, W. W. (1964), Panel Disc. (1959), Ray, I. (1873), Redl (1942), Reinherz (1962), Rosengren (1961), Russell (1949), Schacht & Blacker (1969), Sheeley (1961), Sheffel (1951), Stanton & Schwartz (1949b), Taxel (1953), Toobert et al. (1962), Van Dusen et al. (1963), Worden (1951).

3. *Custodial vs. therapeutic patient care:*
Adams (1961), Adland (1955), Amer. Hosp. Assoc. (1945-

M. (1947), Lewis, A. (1966), Linn (1955a), Macinnes & Macaulay (1963), Mackie (1963), MacKinnon (1963), Maddison (1960), Mahrer (1962), Main (1946), Maine (1947), Mangum (1963), May & Wilkinson (1963), McKerracher (1949), (1961), Mechanick & Nathan (1965), Menninger, W. C. (1936), (1939), (1942), Mercier (1894), von Mering (1957), von Mering & King (1957a), Mishler (1955), Modlin et al. (1958), Montonaro (1964), Moore (1964), Morgan, N. & Johnson (1957), Morgan, R. & Cook (1963), Moss & Boren (1971), Nakagama & Hudsiak (1963), Nat. Assoc. Ment. Health (1946), (1950), (1952), Newcomb (1961), Novey (1960), Opler (1956), Ortega (1962), Osmond (1957), Padula (1960), Peplau (1960), Pepper (1975), Perretz (1960), Pratt et al. (1960), Pratt & Delange (1963), Preston (1948), Pugh & MacMahon (1967), Puthu (1959), Rada (1975), Rapoport & Skellern (1957), Raskin (1958), Rees & Glatt (1956), Reisman (1959), Retznikoff et al. (1959b), Richman & Pinsker (1973), Rinsley (1963), Robbins, C. (1963), Robbins, L. (1963), Robinson, A. M. (1954), Rockefeller (1958), Rothstein (1962), (1966), Rowell (1955), Rudy & Smith (1961), Russell (1949), Sadoff (1975), Schmitt & Gordon (1958), Schreier & Lozito (1963), Schoenberg et al. (1968), Schulberg et al. (1967), Schwartz, A. & Swartzburg (1975), Schwartz, C. (1953), (1957), Schwartz, C. et al. (1951), Schwartz, D. & Waldron (1963), Schwartz, M. (1957a), (1960), Schwartz, M. & Schwartz (1959), (1960), Schwartz, M. & Shockley (1956), Schwartz, M. & Will (1953), Scott, R. (1962), Seale & Watkins (1958), Seitz (1961), (1964), Sewall et al. (1955), Silver & Sines (1963), Silverberg et al. (1964), Simmel (1937), Siradon (1952), Small et al. (1963), Smith, J. et al. (1962), Solt & Walker (1963), Sommer (1958), (1959b), Stanton (1957), Stanton & Schwartz (1954), Stein, W. (1963), Stengel (1948), Stevenson (1942), Stringham (1952), Tallman (1959), Tarwater (1960), Thale (1962), Tietz & Grotjahn (1951), Tischler & Riedel (1973), Todd & Wittkower (1948), Toomey et al. (1961), Tucker & Maxmen (1973), Vaughan & Field (1963), Wales (1960), Walker et al. (1973), Ward (1955), Wayne (1961a), (1961b), Weinstein et al. (1973), Weinstein & Patton (1970), Weintraub (1964), Will, G. (1957), Williams, R. (1957), Williams, T. (1960), Wing (1962),

b. *Psychoanalysts:* Allen (1975), Bandler (1968), Brickman et al. (1966), Brockbank (1971), Ed. Comment (1959f), Feldstein (1939), Freeman, T. (1960), Menninger, W. C. (1939), Robbins, L. (1963), Rosenbaum & Zwerling (1964), Silverberg et al. (1964), Simmel (1937), Stengel (1948), Wadeson (1975), Zwerling (1963).

c. *Psychiatrists:* Coleman (1950), Gynther et al. (1963), Kartus & Schlesinger (1957), Lind & Gralnick (1963), Lubach et al. (1963), Menninger, W. W. (1964), Myers (1951), Panel Disc. (1959), Sheeley (1961), Sheffel (1951), Whitehorn et al. (1953).

d. *Neurologists:* Goody et al. (1960), May (1963), Simon (1961).

e. *Psychologists:* Cowen & Schwartz (1960), Dickson (1949), Gardner, G. (1950).

f. *Social Workers:* Council Soc. Work Educ. (1961), DeWitt (1948), Dickson (1949), Field (1955), GAP (1948a), Hanlon (1961), Harwood (1960), Kantor (1957), Lind & Gralnick (1963), Seefeldt (1964), Singlinger & Faris (1955), White (1943).

g. *Nurses:* Amer. Psychiat. Assoc. (1950b), Ayllon & Michael (1959), Barton (1950), Black, K. (1953), Bush (1960b), Butkiewicz & Fields (1960), Butler & Flood (1962), Curtis, C. (1961), Field (1955), Fields (1960), Fitzsimmons (1950), Graham, E. M. (1964), GAP (1952), (1955), Hunter (1956), Jones, G. & Waldrum (1960), Korson & Hayes (1966), Lipkin & Cohen (1973), Liston (1960), Lubach et al. (1963), McLaughlin (1950), Mereness (1959), Miller (1964), Miller & Sabshin (1963), Mishler (1955), Muller (1950), Myers (1951), Nakagama & Hudsiak (1963), Parloff (1960), Pascoe (1963), Peplau (1956), Pishkin et al. (1961), Render (1947), Robinson, A. et al. (1955), Schmitt & Gordon (1958), Schwartz, C. (1957), Schwartz, M. & Shockley (1956), Singlinger & Faris (1955), Stein, R. (1964), Strune & Hahn (1949), Toomey et al. (1961), Tudor (1952), Wheatley (1963a), (1963b), Will, G. (1957), Williams, J. & Williams (1961).

h. *Activities Therapists:* Folsom (1963), Graham, E. C. & Mullen (1956), Irwin (1963), Jones, M. (1952b), McKerracher (1949), Myers (1951), Pfeffer et al. (1957), Rogers (1963), Sommer (1958), Taggart (1953), Wade (1941), Wolfe (1962).

i. *Psychiatric Aides:* Baer (1952), Ed. Comment (1959c), Eichert (1944), Gerjuoy et al. (1963), Gilbert, D. & Levinson (1957b), Goldman & Lawton (1962), Graham, T. & Zingery (1961), Hall (1957), Hall et al. (1952), Harris & Johnson (1961), Hyde et al. (1956), Johnson, M. & Whitney (1962), Kline (1950), Lewis, G. (1960), Mishler (1955), Morgan, T. & Hall (1950), Nat. Assoc. Ment. Health (1946), (1950), Pearl & Riessman (1966), Pine (1955), Pine & Levinson (1957), Robinson, A. M. (1954), Sterne (1953), Stotsky et al. (1956), Tolor (1962), Williams, J. & Williams (1961).

j. *Volunteers:* Amer. Psychiat. Assoc. (1959), (1964a), Amer. Red Cross (1956), Berry (1963), Conte & Liebes (1960), Doban (1957), Eliasoph (1959), Fechner & Parke (1951), Frank (1949), Haddock & Dundan (1951), Imre (1962), Kantor (1957), Kline (1947), Lerner (1960), McBee & Frank (1950), von Mering (1957), Montonaro (1964), Mounts (1961), Nat. Assoc. Ment. Health (1960), (1961), Overholser (1961), Perkins, M. (1959), Perretz (1960), Phillips, J. (1961), Reinherz (1962), Rockefeller (1958), Rudquist (1962), Seitz (1962), (1963a), Sharp (1953), Shuman (1960), Stetson (1951), Wolff (1960).

k. *Chaplains:* Allport (1943), Bruder (1953), Eberhart (1963), Gluckman (1955), Scully (1945).

l. *Administrative Personnel:* Fitzsimmons (1950), Ryniker (1962).

m. *Maintenance Personnel:* Middleton (1953).

B. Social psychiatric approaches.

1. *Group, milieu, and therapeutic community methods:* Abea & Albright (1960), Abroms (1969), Adland (1955), Almond et al. (1968), Amer. Hosp. Assoc. (1945-75), Anon. (1937), Arthur (1971), (1973), Artiss & Schiff (1969), Baldwin (1963), Banks (1956), Barton (1962c), Bateman & Dunham (1948), Becker (1971), Bonn (1969), Boudwin & Garlington (1959), Carson et al. (1962), Carstairs & Heron (1957), Carty & Breault (1967), Christmas & Davis (1965), Clancey (1959), Clarke (1960), Cone (1964), Conran (1962), Costello & Gazan (1962), Cumming, E. (1962), Cumming, J. & Cumming (1962), Denber (1960a), (1960b), Dinitz et al. (1958), Edelson, M. (1964), Eisen et al. (1963), Fryling & Fryling (1960), Galioni (1952), Galioni et al. (1953), (1957), Garza-Guerrero (1975), Gralnick & D'Elia (1961), Greenblatt (1957a), (1963), Greenblatt et al. (1957), (1965),

Greenblatt & Levinson (1959), Gynther & Gail (1964), Harlow et al. (1956), Hawkins, D. et al. (1973), Herz (1972), Hes & Handler (1961), Horwitz (1968), Irwin (1963), Jackson, J. (1964), Jacoby & McLamb (1959), Jacques (1948), (1957), Jones, M. (1952a), (1952b), (1953), (1956), (1962), (1968a), (1968b), (1973), Jones, M. & Matthews (1956), Jones, M. & Rapoport (1955), (1957), Jones, M. & Tuxford (1963), Kessler (1964), Klemes (1951), Klerman & Mallory (1963), Krammer, C. (1964), Leighton (1955), (1960), Leipold et al. (1964), Lemert (1951), Lewis, A. & Selzer (1972), Luft (1963), Main (1946), Mandelbrote & Freeman (1963), Mann (1959), McGrabee (1961), Menninger, W. C. (1936), Miles (1959), (1962), Murphy, G. & Hunt (1964), Murray & Cohen (1959), Osmond (1957), Panel Disc. (1963), Parloff (1960), Perry & Shea (1957), Pine (1955), Pine & Levinson (1957), Preston (1948), Rabiner et al. (1964), Rapoport (1963), Rapoport & Rapoport (1957), Redlich (1969), Redlich & Astrachan (1969), Rees & Glatt (1955), Rennie (1955), Rioch & Stanton (1953), Robbins, C. (1963), Rosenbaum & Zwerling (1964), Rothaus et al. (1963), Ruesch (1965), (1966), Ruesch & Bareson (1949), Schiff (1969), Schoenberg et al. (1968), Schwartz, C. (1953), Schwartz, C. et al. (1951), Schwartz, M. (1957b), Schwartz, M. & Schwartz (1964), Schwartz, M. & Will (1953), Shattan (1966), Sherif & Sherif (1956), Sherman & Hildreth (1970), Singlinger & Faris (1955), Sletten & Bennett (1963), Small et al. (1963), Smith, H. & Thrasher (1963), Srole & Schrivers (1968), Stainbrook (1955b), Stanton (1957), Strodtbeck & Hare (1954), Thelen (1954), Vail (1964), Vitale (1961), Whitaker & Lieberman (1964), Whitman, R. (1956), Wilkins et al. (1963), Williams, R. (1957), Wilmer (1958a), (1958b), Young (1959), Zeitlyn (1967).
  2. *Open vs. closed wards and hospitals:*
Ackerman, O. et al. (1959), Amer. Hosp. Assoc. (1945-75), Arthur (1971), (1973), Bell (1955), Black, B. (1957), Bonn (1969), Branch (1963a), Branchi et al. (1961), Breggin (1964), Cameron, D. (1950), Cawte & Brown (1962), Clark (1962), Curtis, C. (1961), Delay et al. (1958), Edelson, D. (1960), Ed. Comment (1958), Eisen et al. (1963), Ellenberger (1960), Folkard (1960), Garber (1958), Gilbert, J. (1959), Greenblatt & Lidz (1957), Hacken & Hunt (1959), Hurst (1957), Koltes (1956), Mandelbrote (1958), Mandelbrote & Freeman (1963), Metcalf (1961), Ortega (1962),

(1969), Boquet (1964), Branch (1963b), Bromet (1971), Cameron, D. (1951), Chasin (1967), Cole et al. (1964), Craft (1959), Ferndale (1963), Fisher & Beard (1962), Freeman, H. & Simmons (1958), Freudenthal (1949), Friedman (1963), Garber (1963), Glasscote et al. (1969), Greenblatt (1957a), (1958), Greenblatt et al. (1963), Greenblatt & Lidz (1957), Hargreaves et al. (1962), Keeton (1964), Kimbro & Lemkau (1969), Kramer, B. (1962), Lindsay (1963), Lurie et al. (1956), Naboisek et al. (1957), Odenheimer (1965), Phillips, F. & May (1957), Pitt & Markowe (1963), Pollock (1936), Prince et al. (1973), Rabiner et al. (1962), Reinert et al. (1964), Rothstein (1966), Sampson et al. (1957), Sandall et al. (1975), Shattan (1966), Simmons et al. (1956), Steiman & Hunt (1961), Stokes (1961), Wechsler (1960), (1961), Whitely (1960), Wilson & Bartlett (1955), Wood, P. (1975), Zwerling & Wilder (1962).

6. *Community resources and liaison:*
Amer. Hosp. Assoc. (1945-75), Amer. Med. Assoc. (1964), Arthur (1971), (1973), Beckenstein (1964), Bellak (1964), Black, B. (1957), Blank (1964), Bloomberg (1960), Boquet (1964), Botts (1959), Branch (1963b), Brody, E. (1960), Brown, B. (1963), Brunt (1959), Caplan (1964), Clausen & Radke (1955), Cohen, C. et al. (1975), Coleman (1967), Conte (1960), Cumming, E. & Cumming (1957a), Daniels (1962), Denton (1959), Ed. Comment (1959g), Ewalt (1953), Felix (1961), Felzer et al. (1964), Forstenzer (1961), Freudenthal (1949), Gaede (1962), Garber (1963), Gerty (1964), Goffman (1957), Greenblatt (1957a), (1958), Greenblatt et al. (1963), Greenblatt & Lidz (1957), GAP (1963), (1964), Gussen (1960), Hawkins, N. (1963), Hunt et al. (1961), Jones, M. (1961), Jones, R. (1958), Keskiner et al. (1972), Klopfer et al. (1956), Kolb (1962), Kurland & Nilsson (1961), Lemert (1951), Leyberg (1959), Lurie et al. (1956), Mandelbrote (1959), McLean (1958), Med. Assoc. Ga. (1959), von Mering (1957), Mumford et al. (1971), Naboisek et al. (1957), Nat. Assoc. Ment. Health (1952), Newton (1967), Nurnberger (1961), O'Neill (1960), Opler (1956), Overholser (1942), Parsons (1952), Prince et al. (1953), Rees (1957), Reidy (1964), Ross (1963), Rowland (1939b), Schwartz, C. (1956), Sheeley (1960), Sivadon (1952), Smith, S. et al. (1963), Snow (1962a), Sobin (1959), Stokes (1961), Strauss & Sabshin (1961), Wechsler (1961), Weinberg

(1952), Wilson & Bartlett (1955), Wise et al (1968), Wolfrom et al. (1963).

7. *Community psychiatry: alternatives to hospitalization:*
Amer. Hosp. Assoc. (1945-75), Amer. Psychiat. Assoc. Task Force (1971), Arthur (1971), (1973), Baker, F. & Schulberg (1967), Bandler (1968), Bass & Windle (1972), Berlin (1969), Bindman & Spiegel (1970), Bolman (1968), (1972), Bolman & Westman (1967), Brickman (1967a), (1967b), (1968), (1970), Brockbank (1971), Burrows (1969), Caplan (1961), (1967), Carty & Breault (1967), Christmas & Davis (1965), Coleman (1971), Curtis, W. (1973), Darley & Kenny (1971), Duhl (1967), Duhl & Leopold (1968), Dunham (1965), Fairweather et al. (1969), Farberow (1969), Feldman, S. (1971), Fox & Rappaport (1972), Gardner, E. (1968), Glasscote (1971), Glasscote et al. (1964), (1969), Goldberg, D. (1971), Gray (1968), Hansell (1968), Hart & Bassett (1972), Kanno et al. (1974), Kluger (1970), Kraft et al. (1967), Kramer, M. (1966), Lamb & Goertzel (1971), Leopold (1967), Leopold & Kissick (1970), Lipsius (1973), Lloyd & Wise (1968), Lowenkopf & Zwerling (1971), Macht (1975), Martin, M. (1972), Mumford et al. (1971), Nat. Inst. Ment. Health (1964), Newton (1967), Ozarin et al. (1971), Ozarin & Brown (1965), Pasamanick (1967), Peck et al. (1967), Pumpian-Mindlin (1964), Redlich & Pepper (1968), Reuther (1969), Riessman, C. (1970), Riessman, F. et al. (1964), Riessman, F. & Hallowitz (1967), Rome (1965), Ryan, W. (1969), Sabshin (1969), Sainsbury (1969), Schaffer & Myers (1954), Scherl (1966), Scherl & English (1969), Schwartz, R. (1969), Smith, C. (1971), Srole & Schrijvers (1968), Strickler (1965), Stubblebine & Decker (1971), Thomson (1970), Thomson & Bell (1969), Torrey (1969), Wachpress (1972), Wadeson (1975), Williams, R. & Ozarin (1968), Wise et al. (1968), Wolford et al. (1972), Yolles et al. (1967), Zwerling (1963), Zwerling & Coleman (1959).

C. Training and research.
1. *Training programs:*
Amer. Hosp. Assoc. (1945-75), Amer. Psychiat. Assoc. (1964a), Argyris (1962), Artiss & Schiff (1969), Barchilon (1964), Bartlett & Aurnhammer (1957), Beisser et al. (1959), Bellak et al. (1963), Borsch (1963), Bosworth (1959), Bovard (1951), Braceland (1962), Bradford (1953),

(1961), (1963), Bradford et al. (1964), Bravos (1959), Briggs
& Wood (1956), Brody, D. et al. (1960), Butkiewicz & Fields
(1960), Connery (1951), Council Soc. Work Educ. (1961),
Council State Govts. (1953), Curry (1959), Daniels (1962),
Davies (1962), Dickson (1949), Ed. Comment (1959c),
(1959f), Eichert (1944), Eisenberg (1973), Felzer et al.
(1964), Fleming & Hamburg (1958), Freeman, T. (1960),
Gaede (1962), Gaitonde (1963), Gertz (1963), Gold-
berg, N. & Hyde (1954), Greenblatt (1957a), Greenblatt
et al. (1957), GAP (1955), Hall et al. (1951), Ham (1961),
Harris & Johnson (1961), Hoch & Rado (1961), Horwitz
(1968), Johnson, M. & Whitney (1962), Jones, M. (1962),
Kantor (1957), Lewis, G. (1960), Linn (1955a), Luft (1963),
Masserman (1963), McDermott & Maretzki (1975), Miles
(1959), (1962), Mishler (1955), Modlin (1951), Moran &
Leopold (1963), Morgan, T. & Hall (1950), Overholser
(1942), Pascoe (1963), Perkins, G. (1952), Pumpian-
Mindlin (1964), Redlich & Astrachan (1969), Rothaus et al.
(1963), Ryan (1964), Seitz (1961), (1962), (1963a), (1963b),
(1964), Sheeley (1960), Sherman & Hildreth (1970), Silver
& Sines (1963), Silverberg et al. (1964), Simmel (1937), Solt
& Walker (1963), Stein, R. (1964), Stewart et al. (1963),
Taggart (1953), West (1973), Whitehorn et al. (1953).

2. *Research programs:*
Amer. Hosp. Assoc. (1945-75), Amer. Psychiat. Assoc. Task
Force (1971), Baker, F. (1966), Becker (1967), (1975),
Brody, E. (1964), Cancro (1969), (1970), Carter (1959),
Council State Govts. (1953), Davis, J. E. (1957), Dinitz et al.
(1961), Dykens (1964), Ekman (1961), Etzioni (1960),
Framo & Adlerstein (1961), Glick (1975), Glueck (1963),
Greenblatt (1958), (1962), Greenblatt et al. (1957), GAP
(1954), Hawkins, N. (1961), Kahn, M. et al. (1963), Kandel
& Williams (1964), Kramer, M. (1957), Kurland (1962),
Landy (1961), Lasky (1962), Levinson (1957), Lewinsohn &
Nichols (1964), Lubach et al. (1963), Luezki (1958),
Morimoto (1955), Noroian (1962), Retznikoff et al. (1959a),
Robinson, A. et al. (1955), Rosenberg et al. (1962), Sabshin
(1962), Schreier & Lozito (1963), Simpson & Kline (1962),
Soc. Sci. Inst. (1961), Sokolov (1960), Stanton (1957),
Strodtbeck & Hare (1954), Tarjan (1964), Vitale (1961),
Wechsler et al. (1962).

3. *The consultant team approach:*
Amer. Hosp. Assoc. (1945-75), Blank (1964), Daniels (1962), Denton (1959), Dykens et al. (1964), Hutt et al. (1947), Linn (1955a), Perkins, G. (1952), Seitz et al. (1963), Stewart et al. (1963).